THIRD EDITION

REFRACTION

A PROGRAMMED TEXT

Robert D. Reinecke, M.D.

Department of Ophthalmology
Jefferson Medical College
Wills Eye Hospital
Philadelphia, Pennsylvania

Robert J. Herm, M.D.

Keene Clinic
Keene, New Hampshire

APPLETON-CENTURY-CROFTS/Norwalk, Connecticut

0-8385-8300-8

Notice: The authors and publisher of this volume have taken care that the information
and recommendations contained herein are accurate and compatible with the standards generally
accepted at the time of publication.

Copyright © 1983 by Appleton-Century-Crofts
A Publishing Division of Prentice-Hall, Inc.

83 84 85 86 87 88 / 10 9 8 7 6 5 4 3 2 1

Prentice-Hall International, Inc., London
Prentice-Hall of Australia, Pty. Ltd., Sydney
Prentice-Hall Canada, Inc.
Prentice-Hall of India Private Limited, New Delhi
Prentice-Hall of Japan, Inc., Tokyo
Prentice-Hall of Southeast Asia (Pte.) Ltd., Singapore
Whitehall Books Ltd., Wellington, New Zealand
Editora Prentice-Hall do Brasil Ltda., Rio de Janeiro

Library of Congress Cataloging in Publication Data

Reinecke, Robert D.
  Refraction.

  Includes index.
    1. Eye—Accomodation and refraction—Programmed
instruction. I. Herm, Robert J. II. Title.
[DNLM: 1. Refraction, Ocular—Programmed texts.
WW 18 R366r]
RE925.R43 1983   617.7′55′077   83-2840
ISBN 0-8385-8300-8

Design: Jean M. Sabato

PRINTED IN THE UNITED STATES OF AMERICA

This book is dedicated to
Betsey Herm
and
Mary Reinecke

Preface

Our aspiration for this book remains unaltered in this third edition—namely to assist the neophyte refractionist over the early hurdles in the rather painful race to become a reasonably skilled refractionist. The results of the first two editions were gratifying. The third edition is further refined in the specifics of the frames, which, we hope, makes it clearer and less confusing than the original text. Some major changes in ophthalmology are reflected in some of the new subjects covered, such as pseudophakia, soft contact lenses of better quality, and automated refractometers. We recognize that the student of refraction is learning a great many other subjects at this time, but refraction is a daily problem of the first order in patient care. If this text makes the task easier through this relatively simple format, you and your patients may be grateful. We urge you to read fairly rapidly through the book, repeating the process from time to time. The subsequent readings proceed much faster and become more meaningful as you look back at real problems in refraction which you have failed to solve, or perhaps even have created. The subject may appear difficult to you at this point, but several years from now you will be convinced that "there is nothing to it." If this edition can make you say this sooner, your time and ours will have been well spent.

Robert D. Reinecke, M.D.
Robert J. Herm, M.D.

Contents

To the Student

This programmed text is designed to teach you its subject in an effective manner. Unlike an ordinary textbook, this program is set up so that you will learn on a step-by-step basis by making an *active* response to a question and then immediately comparing your answer with a printed answer on the next page.

This method of teaching is called "programmed instruction," and depends on the careful analysis of the information given and its presentation in a sequence of *frames*. Each frame provides new information to which you respond by answering a question, completing a sentence, or otherwise using the information you have just received. Checking against the correct answer allows you to evaluate your progress immediately. For the program to be successful, it is important that you actually *write* all the required responses. Most answers will come easily, but if you go along merely "thinking" your answers, you will not remember what you learn, and you will not grasp later material. Remember, the program will teach effectively only if the proper order of items is followed and every answer is written *before* referring to the correct answer on the following page.

Proceed through the program in the following manner:

1. Start at frame 1 at the top of page 1, and after reading the frame turn to page 3.

2. Read the question in frame 2 at the top of page 3.

3. Write your answer in the blank space provided in the frame.

4. Turn to page 5 and compare your written answer with the printed answer in the small answer frame 2 in the left-hand corner of the page.

5. Continue on page 5, answering the question in frame 3 and checking your answer on page 7. Go on to the next frame in the same way. Be sure to go through the frames in numerical order.

6. After you have answered all the frames in the top layer on the right-hand pages, return to page 1 and continue on the second row of frames. Go through all the right-hand pages this way.

7. When you have completed all the frames on the right-hand pages, turn to page 2, and follow the same procedure for the left-hand pages.

From time to time, the program will refer to illustrative reference material, which is included in the Appendix at the end of the book. These references to the Appendix will appear in a form such as the following: (See Fig. 1, p. 347.). When you reach such a reference, turn to the appropriate figure in the Appendix as instructed in the program.

1.

PART I

NEUTRALIZATION OF LENSES AND
THE MEASUREMENT OF VISUAL ACTIVITY

(Turn to page 3.)

---

173. The amplitude of accommodation is typically approximately equal in the two eyes. A patient with an amplitude of accommodation of 8.00 D in the right eye will probably have an amplitude of _____ D in the left eye.

---

345. Occasionally you may wish to use only spheres to refract an astigmatic eye. A stenopaic slit as pictured may be used. If the slit were held at 180 degrees and the patient required a +2.00 D sphere, and if the slit were held at 90 degrees and the patient required a +1.00 D sphere the patient's refractive error would be

_____.
(sphere, cylinder, and axis)

Remember the power of a cylinder is 90 degrees from its axis.

+2.00 = Refractive error   +1.00 = Refractive error

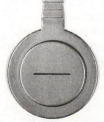
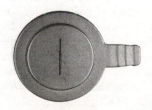

Position "A"   Position "B"

517. Patient A is directed to look at the Lancaster-Regan dial 20 feet away with a −0.75 sphere before the right eye and an occluder before the left. The photograph shows how the dial appears to patient A. By walking to the chart and holding a pointer parallel to various lines, you determine that the blackest and clearest lines indicate the axis of the correcting minus cylinder to be _____ degrees. *(Record on data sheet; see Fig. 7.)*

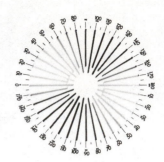

---

689. The adequacy of cycloplegia can only be determined by measuring _____.

---

861. As a clinical problem aniseikonia is rarely recognized and rarely clinically significant. Its measurement is time consuming and its correcting lenses expensive and cosmetically inferior. If aniseikonia due to anisometropia is anticipated, it is frequently minimized by undercorrecting one eye. The incidence of clinically significant aniseikonia is unknown, but a measurable amount should be found in 20 to 30 percent of spectacle wearers.

Aniseikonia due to anisometropia can be minimized by _____.

2. The eye is an optical system which forms discrete images on the retina. Any defect in this optical system may throw the image out of focus. Ophthalmic lenses may correct such defects. The measurement of these optical defects is called refraction.

This programmed course is designed to help you acquire the basic skills in _____ .

---

173. 8.00 D

---

174. Accommodation changes inversely with age. The first reasonably accurate study of the relationship between accommodative amplitude and age was published in 1912 by Duane. Duane's graph relates the decrease in amplitude of accommodation to _____ .

---

345. $+2.00 - 1.00 \times 180$ (or $+1.00 + 1.00 \times 90$)

---

346. If the radius of curvature is uniform in each separate meridian (although the radii of the meridians may differ), the astigmatism is termed regular. If there are many radii in one meridian, such as a scarred cornea might have, the astigmatism is termed irregular. To correct irregular astigmatism, the irregularities in the surface must be corrected or covered. Irregular astigmatism would probably be corrected by (1) _____ , while regular astigmatism is usually corrected with (2) _____ .

517. *(Be sure to record 25 degrees on Fig. 7.)*

518. Continuing with the refraction of patient A, OD, dial No. 2 is turned so that one line is at (1) _____ degrees and the other line is at (2) _____ degrees.

689. residual accommodation

690. A patient over age 10 will generally have a satisfactorily low residual accommodation for cycloplegic refraction with the use of the short-acting drugs (1) _____ or (2) _____ .

861. undercorrecting one eye

862. Some of the intolerance of patients to spectacles is a result of magnification of retinal images. Aberrations of lenses are another cause of spectacle intolerance, as are prismatic effects. Two causes of intolerance to spectacles in addition to magnification of retinal images are (1) _____ and (2) _____ .

4

2. refraction

---

3. The properties of ophthalmic lenses will be considered first. These properties will be used as basic tools in measuring the refractive state of the eye, that is, in the procedure called _____.

---

174. age (increasing age)

---

175. Duane's graph relates (1) _____ to (2) _____.

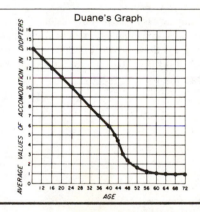

Duane's Graph

---

346. (1) contact lenses
(2) cylindrical spectacle lenses

---

347. Astigmatism caused by irregular refracting surfaces is called _____.

518. (1) 25 \
   (2) 115 / either order

---

519. Patient A is directed to observe dial No. 2 with OD through a −0.75 sphere in the trial frame and sees that the line at _____ degrees on the dial is the blacker and clearer.

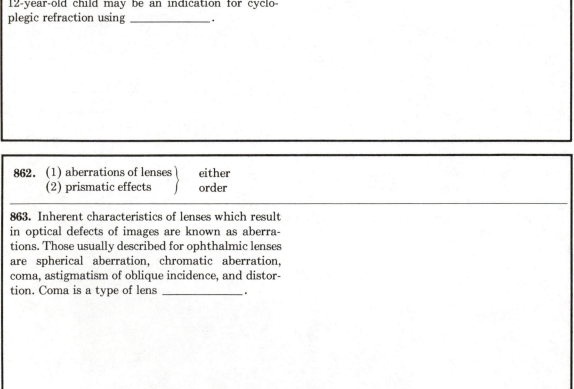

---

690. (1) cyclopentolate \
   (2) tropicamide / either order

---

691. The darker the patient's iris in color, the more effective the cycloplegic which must be used for refraction. A deep brown iris pigmentation in a 12-year-old child may be an indication for cycloplegic refraction using _____.

---

862. (1) aberrations of lenses \
   (2) prismatic effects / either order

---

863. Inherent characteristics of lenses which result in optical defects of images are known as aberrations. Those usually described for ophthalmic lenses are spherical aberration, chromatic aberration, coma, astigmatism of oblique incidence, and distortion. Coma is a type of lens _____.

6

3. refraction

---

4. The term **spherical** refers to a lens that does either one of two things: either it converges parallel rays of light passing through it to a point focus, or it diverges them so that they appear to come from a point source. The lens in the diagram brings parallel rays of light to a point focus indicating that it is a _____ converging lens.

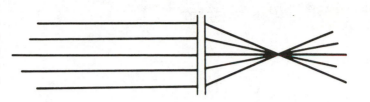

---

175. (1) amplitude of accommodation ⎱ either
(2) age ⎰ order

---

176. The average amplitude of accommodation of a child 8 years old is about 14.00 D. At age 35, it is about 7.00 D. Refer to Duane's graph. At what age is the average amplitude of accommodation 10.00 D?

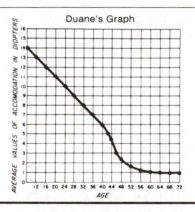

Duane's Graph

---

347. irregular astigmatism

---

348. Irregular astigmatism can be corrected only by substituting a new surface. The only practical means of achieving this is to do a corneal graft of the deformed cornea or use a contact lens, which in effect creates a new surface.

Irregular astigmatism (can/cannot) be corrected with cylindrical spectacle lenses.

519. 115

---

520. With the blacker and clearer line on dial No. 2 at 115 degrees, minus cylinders will be placed before the eye at axis _____ degrees.

---

691. atropine

---

692. The cycloplegic drug with the longest effect on accommodation is _____.

---

863. aberration

---

864. Spherical aberration results from the fact that rays of light parallel to the axis of the lens are focused closer to the lens the further from the axis they enter it. This causes a point object to be focused to an image symmetrically blurred around the axis of the lens. Symmetrical blurring of the image of a point source around the axis of a lens is known as _____.

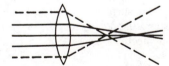

4. spherical

---

5. Spherical lenses may be convex or concave. Convex lenses converge rays of light, and concave lenses diverge rays of light. The lens diagrammed is a _____ spherical lens.

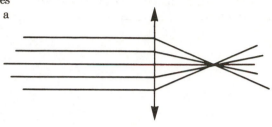

---

176. 24

---

177. Refer to Duane's graph of accommodation versus age. A patient's amplitude of accommodation is 3.00 D. About what age is the average patient with this amplitude?

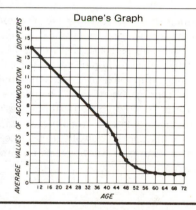

---

348. cannot

---

349. Irregular astigmatism is usually corneal in nature but may be refractive due to different indices of refraction in different portions of the crystalline lens. Will a contact lens correct irregular astigmatism of the crystalline lens?

520. 25

---

521. Sets of trial lenses provide pairs of lenses of each power. The sign of the cylinders and spheres is indicated on the _____.

---

692. atropine

---

693. A combination of topical drugs has been found to yield adequate relaxation in all but the unusual patient. The combination consists of first a drop of topical anesthetic such as .5 percent proparacaine, followed by one drop each of 1 percent tropicamide, and 2 percent cyclopentolate. The purpose of the anesthetic is twofold; first, it diminishes the discomfort of the subsequent drops and second, it allows better ocular penetration of the cycloplegics. In most cases (atropine/the above combination) will be preferred.

---

864. spherical aberration

---

865. Spherical aberration can be minimized by grinding one surface of a lens aspherically. The higher the power of the lens, the greater the spherical aberration. Significant spherical aberration can therefore be expected with aphakic lenses and can be minimized by the use of _____ lenses.

5. convex

---

6. Convex lenses are plus lenses. This is easy to remember if you think of convex lenses as bulging, almost as if something were added; convex lenses are therefore called (1) _____ lenses.

Concave lenses, on the other hand, look as if they had been hollowed out—like a cave—and as if something had been subtracted. Therefore, concave lenses are called (2) _____ lenses.

---

177. 46

---

178. Where is the near point of accommodation of an emmetrope whose amplitude of accommodation is 5.00 D?

---

349. No

---

350. The retina normally provides a smooth surface for images. If the retina is raised, as with tumor or inflammation, it may not be uniformly elevated and _____ may result.

521. handles

---

522. The handles of cylindrical lenses in the trial sets are designed so that the left lens in each pair is to be used before the patient's right eye and the right lens of each pair before the patient's left eye. To neutralize the astigmatic error of patient A's right eye, cylindrical lenses on the _____ side of the trial set will be used.

---

693. the above combination

---

694. Cycloplegic refractions in adults are generally done with short-acting drugs for the convenience of the patient. The two most effective drugs in this category are (1) _____ and (2) _____ .

---

865. aspheric

---

866. Coma is a variety of spherical aberration affecting rays of light obliquely incident to a lens. It occurs, therefore, off the axis of the lens and is asymmetrical, giving a blurred image resembling a comet. Coma differs from spherical aberration in its (1) _____ and by the fact that it affects rays of light passing through the lens (2) _____ .

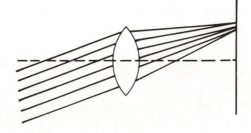

6. (1) plus
   (2) minus

7. Convex lenses are called "plus" lenses and concave lenses are called "minus" lenses. The lens diagrammed is a (plus/ minus) spherical lens.

---

178. 20 cm (or 8 inches)

179. A hyperopic eye requires plus power for correction. Hyperopia may be totally or partially corrected by the eye's own _____.

---

350. astigmatism

351. Approximately 0.25 D of astigmatism is considered physiologic if it is corrected with +0.25 C axis 90 degrees. This astigmatism usually increases slightly with age and has been attributed to the lids squeezing the cornea, causing the vertical meridian to have a smaller radius (hence more power) than the horizontal. This is called **with the rule** astigmatism. At what axis should a minus cylinder be placed to correct with the rule astigmatism?

522. left

---

523. When a cylinder is placed in a trial frame, it is placed in a front cell so that the axis may be accurately varied. The line marking the axis of a trial cylinder is aligned with the appropriate degree mark on the front surface by turning the wheel located on the _____.

---

694. (1) cyclopentolate ⎞ either
     (2) tropicamide ⎠ order

---

695. Cycloplegia alters the normal accommodative-convergence relationship, and it eliminates the opportunity of studying the patient's normal accommodative habits. Except in young children, therefore, it is usually necessary to perform a pre- or postcycloplegic refraction, including muscle tests. Subjective refraction and muscle testing following accommodative recovery from a cycloplegic refraction is known as _____ refraction.

---

866. (1) asymmetry (or image)
     (2) obliquely

---

867. Aspheric lenses are expensive and hence their use is reserved for high-powered lenses. A less effective but more practical method of reducing spherical aberration in lenses of average power is bending the lens. Which lens (A/B) could be expected to produce less spherical aberration?

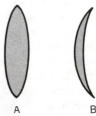

A   B

14

7. plus

---

8. The amount of divergence or convergence ability a lens possesses is called its **power.** Power is measured in diopters. A lens which focuses parallel rays of light 1 m from the lens has a power of 1 diopter. The formula is written:

$$D \text{ (diopter)} = \frac{1}{f \text{ (focal length in meters)}}.$$

The power of the lens in the diagram is _____ .

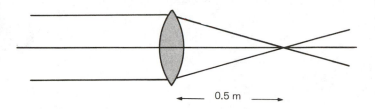

0.5 m

---

179. accommodation

---

180. Hyperopia is a refractive error of insufficient plus power in the eye.

As long in life as accommodation is active, a certain amount of hyperopia is corrected by physiological tone of the ciliary muscles. The portion of hyperopia so corrected is termed latent hyperopia. The remaining hyperopia is termed manifest hyperopia. Total hyperopia is the sum of (1) _____ hyperopia and (2) _____ hyperopia.

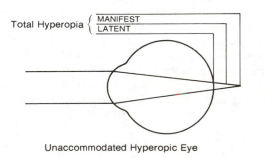

Total Hyperopia { MANIFEST / LATENT

Unaccommodated Hyperopic Eye

---

351. 180 degrees

---

352. Against the rule astigmatism occurs when the horizontal meridian has more power. A minus cylinder at what axis will correct against the rule astigmatism?

523. outer side of the lens carrier
   (or similar wording)

---

524. To maintain the posterior focal line of the conoid of Sturm anterior to the retina, plus spheres must be placed in the trial frame as minus cylinders are added. For each additional -0.50 D cylinder, $+$ _____ sphere is added.

---

695. postcycloplegic

---

696. Postcycloplegic or precycloplegic refraction includes a brief verification of astigmatic error and, more importantly, in the case of hyperopia, a determination of the latent component. A hyperopic patient will not comfortably wear a distance correction which attempts to correct even as little as 0.25 D of his latent hyperopia. Postcycloplegic refraction is necessary in hyperopes to determine how much of the total hyperopia is _____.

---

867. B

---

868. Chromatic aberration occurs because each wavelength is refracted to a slightly different degree and results in color fringes around white light.
   Color fringes around white light seen through spectacles are a sign of _____.

8. 2 D

9. A + or − written before the dioptric power of a lens indicates whether a lens converges or diverges light. A plus lens converges light and is called a convex lens. A minus lens (1) _____ light and is called a (2) _____ lens.

---

180. (1) latent ⎫ either
　　　 (2) manifest ⎭ order

---

181. Manifest hyperopia is divided between absolute and facultative hyperopia. Absolute hyperopia is that amount of hyperopia which cannot be corrected by accommodation. If a 6.00 D hyperopic eye can correct only 4.00 D by accommodation, the remaining 2.00 D of hyperopia is termed _____ hyperopia.

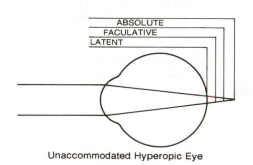

Unaccommodated Hyperopic Eye

---

352. 90 degrees

---

353. With the rule astigmatism has been found to interfere less with the visual acuity than against the rule astigmatism. Which patient, A or B, will be most likely to need the indicated lens to correct vision?

- A: plano + 1.00 × 90
- B: plano + 1.00 × 180

524. 0.25 D

525. A +0.25 D sphere and −0.50 D cylinder axis 25 degrees are added to the −0.75 D sphere already in the trial frame before OD of patient A, and you determine that he sees dial No. 2 as pictured in Figure B. With only the −0.75 D sphere before the eye it appeared as in Figure A. This indicates that the astigmatic error is (undercorrected/overcorrected).

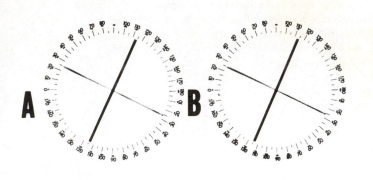

696. latent (or manifest)

697. In the case of patients who are too young or too intellectually impaired to cooperate for the purpose of subjective verification of retinoscopy, it is necessary to prescribe on the basis of retinoscopy alone. When subjective refraction is not possible, glasses may be prescribed from _____ findings.

868. chromatic aberration

869. Chromatic dispersion is the separation of white light into its spectrum by unequal refraction of various wavelengths. Chromatic aberration can be reduced by utilizing glass with a low chromatic dispersion in spectacle manufacture. This will decrease the difference in _____ between different wavelengths of light.

9. (1) diverges
    (2) concave

---

10. The focal length of a minus lens is measured as the distance between the lens and the point from which rays of light that reached the lens as parallel appear to diverge after passing through the lens. The power of the minus lens in the diagram is

_____ .

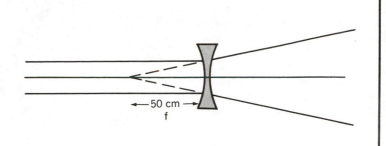

←—50 cm —→
f

---

181. absolute

---

182. Facultative hyperopia is that amount of hyperopia which can be corrected by an effort of accommodation over and above the accommodation provided by physiological tone of the ciliary muscles. If a 6.00 D hyperopic eye has 1.00 D of latent hyperopia and 1.00 D of absolute hyperopia, the remainder is termed _____ hyperopia.

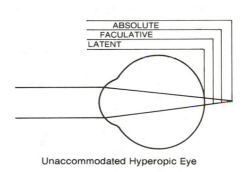

ABSOLUTE
FACULATIVE
LATENT

Unaccommodated Hyperopic Eye

---

353. B

---

354. For each of the listed astigmatic corrections check whether the patient has with the rule or against the rule astigmatism.

	With the Rule	Against the Rule
(1) plano + 2.00 × 90		
(2) plano + 1.00 × 180		
(3) plano − 1.50 × 180		
(4) plano − 2.00 × 90		

525. undercorrected

526. A +0.75 D sphere and −1.50 D cylinder axis 25 degrees are added to the −0.75 D sphere in the trial frame before OD of patient A, and dial No. 2 appears to him as pictured in Figure B. With only the −0.75 D sphere before the eye it appeared as in Figure A. The astigmatic error is _____.

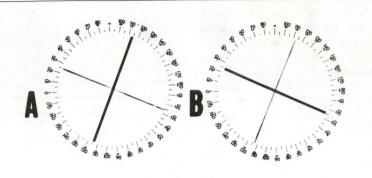

697. retinoscopy

698. If prescribing is to be based only on retinoscopy and a cycloplegic has been used, an arbitrary decision must be made as to how much hyperopia is latent. In hyperopic patients for whom glasses will be prescribed on the basis of cycloplegic retinoscopy, allowance must be made for _____ hyperopia when prescribing.

869. refraction

870. Obliquely incident rays are not only subject to coma but also result in a truly astigmatic focus with two focal lines and a circle of least confusion. This aberration is called astigmatism of oblique incidence. A line connecting the circles of least confusion, resulting from different degrees of obliquity of incidence, is not the theoretical focal plane but is curved symmetrically. Undesirable astigmatic foci are the result of the lens aberration called _____.

10. 2 D

---

11. A $+4.00$ D lens is a (1) (convex/concave) lens with a focal length of (2) _____ cm.

---

182. facultative

---

183. Manifest hyperopia is divided between absolute and facultative. Absolute hyperopia is that amount of hyperopia which cannot be corrected by accommodation. An eye which cannot accommodate to correct all its hyperopia requires a lens to improve the distance visual acuity to normal. The power of the lens necessary to provide normal visual acuity for this eye is a measure of its _____ hyperopia.

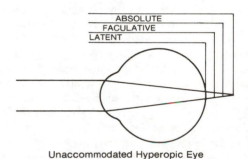

ABSOLUTE
FACULATIVE
LATENT

Unaccommodated Hyperopic Eye

---

354. (1) With the rule   (3) With the rule
(2) Against the rule   (4) Against the rule

---

355. If the axis of the correcting cylinder is other than near 90 degrees or 180 degrees (other than with or against the rule) then the astigmatism is called oblique astigmatism.

Write the type of astigmatism

(1) $+2.00 - 1.00 \times 90$ _____ astigmatism
(2) $+3.00 - 2.00 \times 45$ _____ ″
(3) $+2.00 - 1.50 \times 180$ _____ ″
(4) $+1.00 + 2.00 \times 180$ _____ ″
(5) $-2.00 + 2.00 \times 90$ _____ ″
(6) $-2.00 - 3.00 \times 135$ _____ ″

526. overcorrected
   (or equivalent term)

527. A $+0.50$ D sphere and -1.00 D cylinder axis 25 degrees is added to the -0.75 D sphere in the trial frame before OD of patient A and dial No. 2 looks to him as pictured. The astigmatic error has been _____ .

698. latent

699. The more effective the cycloplegia the greater is the arbitrary allowance for latent hyperopia if prescribing is to be based on cycloplegic retinoscopy only. A hyperopic child who has been retinoscoped following the full cycloplegic dose of atropine will, in the absence of strabismus, be prescribed spectacles with spheres 2.00 D weaker than the net retinoscopy. If a weaker cycloplegic, such as homatropine, were used, less accommodation would be relaxed; therefore, (more/less) than the 2 D allowance for the atropine retinoscopy would be made.

870. astigmatism of oblique incidence

871. If a lens is tipped, rays of light which would otherwise be parallel to its axis will enter the lens _____ .

11. (1) convex
    (2) 25

12. The lens drawn is a (1) (convex/concave) lens with a power of (2) _____ D.

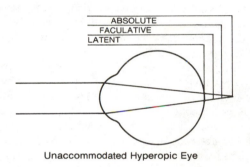

←—33.33 cm—→

183. absolute

184. With absolute hyperopia corrected, the visual acuity of an eye is 20/20. As additional plus power is added to the correction, vision remains 20/20 as accommodation relaxes. Thereafter additional plus power results in decreased visual acuity since latent hyperopia cannot be measured without drugs. The plus power which can be added to the correction after visual acuity becomes 20/20 until it begins to decrease (without drugs) is a measure of the _____ hyperopia.

ABSOLUTE
FACULATIVE
LATENT

Unaccommodated Hyperopic Eye

355. (1) against the rule   (4) against the rule
    (2) oblique   (5) with the rule
    (3) with the rule   (6) oblique

356. Tilting a lens produces a toric surface to incident light and creates astigmatism, so that when the crystalline lens of the eye is tilted, or partly subluxated, astigmatism will result. If the lens is clear, this astigmatism will probably be (regular/irregular).

527. neutralized (or corrected)

---

528. With the eye fogged, a −1.00 D cylinder has made the lines on dial No. 2 appear equally (1) _____ and (2) _____, indicating neutralization of the astigmatic error.

---

699. less

---

700. In hyperopic children without strabismus if noncyloplegic subjective verification of retinoscopy is not feasible, the allowance for latent hyperopia using atropine is 2.00 D; using the combination of proparacaine, cyclopentolate, and tropicamide 2.00 D; using cyclopentolate, scopolamine, or tropicamide 1.50 D; and using homotropine 1.00 D. A 3-year-old child has been retinoscoped following use of cyclopentolate alone with the net retinoscopy OD + 6.00 − 3.00 × 170. The lens prescribed for OD will be _____.

---

871. obliquely

---

872. Obliquely incident rays give rise to the aberrations of coma and _____.

12. (1) concave

(2) 3 (or −3.00)

---

13. Spherical lenses include concave and convex lenses. A lens which focuses parallel rays of light to a point or diverges parallel rays of light so they appear to come from a point source is called a _____ lens.

---

184. facultative

---

185. Myopia is a refractive error of too much plus power. Because of the adverse effect on visual acuity, myopes do not accommodate when viewing distant objects. If a 3.00 D myope attempts to see an object at 20 feet without his correction, what accommodation will be utilized?

---

356. regular

---

357. The ciliary muscle contracts equally in all meridians; if it did not, _____ would be produced when the eye accommodated.

528. (1) black ⎫ either
(2) clear (or blurred) ⎭ order

529. The power of lenses before OD of patient A, with the astigmatism neutralized and the eye still fogged, totals $-0.25 - 1.00 \times 29$ *(record on Fig. 7)*. The visual acuity is 20/40. The conoid of Sturm has been eliminated; thus a (1) _____ focus is present which is (2) _____ to the retina.

700. $+4.50 - 3.00 \times 170$

701. The process of reducing spherical power is known as cutting the sphere. If atropine is used for cycloplegia and postcycloplegic examination is not feasible, the sphere will be cut _____ before prescribing for a hyperopic child without strabismus.

872. astigmatism of oblique incidence

873. The pantoscopic tilt of spectacles is generally a compromise between the degree of tilt needed for entry of rays parallel to the axis of the lens with eyes in the reading position and that needed for parallelism when gaze is directed to far distances. This compromise is necessary to minimize the aberrations called (1) _____ and (2) _____ .

13. spherical

---

14. The power of a lens is measured in (1) _____ and is the reciprocal of its (2) _____ measured in meters.

---

185. none

---

186. Accommodation results in increased plus power. The distance vision of an uncorrected myope will be _____ if he accommodates.

---

357. astigmatism (regular astigmatism)

---

358. Symptoms of astigmatism vary greatly from patient to patient. Many patients will tolerate great or small amounts of astigmatism without difficulty, their only complaint being poor vision with larger degrees of astigmatism. Smaller amounts of astigmatism, 0.75 D to 2.00 D, may cause asthenopic symptoms as the patient constantly refocuses from one end of the conoid of Sturm to the other. What would you expect a patient with 4.00 D astigmatism to have as his chief complaint?

529. (1) point
(2) anterior

530. The point focus anterior to the retina is moved toward the retina by the addition of _____ spheres in 0.25 D steps.
(sign)

701. 2.00 D

702. If scopolamine, cyclopentolate, or tropicamide are used for cycloplegia, the sphere will be cut (1) _____ D; if homatropine is used, the sphere will be cut (2) _____ before prescribing for a hyperopic child without strabismus.

873. (1) astigmatism of oblique incidence } either
(2) coma } order

874. The angle a spectacle lens makes with the temple of the frame is known as _____.

14. (1) diopters
(2) focal length

(Use a regular trial lens set for this frame.)

15. Observe your trial lens case. Note that it is divided into at least five compartments, labeled Cylindrical Concave, Cylindrical Convex, Spherical Concave, Spherical _____, and Accessories.

---

186. worsened (or decreased)

---

187. At 33.33 cm an uncorrected 3.00 D myope will use no accommodation. If a 3.00 D myope attempts near work without correction at 20 cm, how much accommodation must be used?

---

358. poor vision

---

359. It is frequently perplexing to correct an astigmatism of a large amount in a young person and find the patient's vision improved only slightly. The new corrected image apparently causes difficulty in interpretation which needs only time to resolve. The full astigmatic error correction should be given a young person. When the vision is retested after a few months of continuous wearing of the astigmatic correction, the improvement in visual acuity is usually gratifying.

Patient is age eight. Refractive error = +3.00 − 3.00 × 180 OU.* Best vision = 20/70. No previous glasses. No pathology.

(1) What lens would you prescribe?
(2) May vision improve to 20/20?

*OU means "in each eye" or "with both eyes."

530. minus

---

531. When -0.75 D sphere has been added to the lenses before OD of patient A, his visual acuity has been improved to 20/15. The total power of lenses before OD is now _____. *(Refer to Fig. 7, your last entry.)*

---

702. (1) 1.50
(2) 1.00 D

---

703. In the case of myopia, if glasses are to be prescribed on the basis of cycloplegic retinoscopy alone, the net retinoscopy may be prescribed without alteration. This is because myopes do not (1) _____ at distance. If a patient has a net retinoscopy of -2.50 D OD under atropine cycloplegia, (2) _____ D concave lens OD will be prescribed.

---

874. pantoscopic tilt

---

875. The higher the lens power, the greater the astigmatism of oblique incidence. When retinoscoping high myopes or aphakic patients, if lenses are tipped, significant _____ can be induced.

30

15. Convex

(Use a regular trial lens set for this frame.)

16. The numbers dividing the columns of the lens case indicate the power of the lenses in the slot on each side. The 0.50 in the compartment labeled Spherical Convex indicates the lenses in the adjacent slots have a _____ of 0.50 D.

---

187. 2.00 D

---

188. An eye has a visual acuity of 20/40 uncorrected. A +1.00 D lens improves the vision to 20/20 and it remains 20/20 with a +1.75 D lens. A +2.00 D lens reduces the vision to 20/25. The manifest hyperopia is (1) _____ D, of which (2) _____ D is absolute and (3) _____ D is facultative.

---

359. (1) +3.00 − 3.00 × 180 OU
 (2) Yes (not uncommon)

---

360. Correction of large errors of astigmatism in adults may present difficulties. If a full astigmatic correction (which has not been worn previously) is given, the change of images may be intolerable. It is usual to warn patients of visual distortions if they are about to wear a large astigmatic correction for the first time. Cylindrical lenses cause (less/more) distortion than similarly powered spherical lenses?

531. $-1.00 -1.00 \times 25$ *(Record this answer in ap-propriate space on Fig. 7.)*

532. A -0.25 D sphere is added to the final correc-tion before OD of patient A. The visual acu-ity remains 20/15. The patient has begun to
_____ .

703. (1) accommodate
(2) -2.50

704. The decision as to whether or not to prescribe a new correction for a patient depends on his visual requirements and symptoms. The two factors dictating the prescription of a new correction for a patient are (1) _____ and (2)
_____ .

875. astigmatism (or astigmatism of oblique inci-dence)

876. During retinoscopy of eyes with high refrac-tive errors, special care must be taken that the retinoscope, center of the lenses, and visual axis are all aligned. If this is not done, erroneous
_____ may be noted.
(type refractive error)

16. power

(Use a regular trial lens set for this frame.)

17. The handle of a lens in a trial case indicates the power and sign of the lens. The power is printed on the sign cut into the handle. Remove the lens from the slot labeled Spherical Concave 1.00. Sketch the handle.

---

188. (1) 1.75
   (2) 1.00
   (3) 0.75

---

189. As accommodation decreases with aging, all hyperopia, latent and facultative, gradually becomes absolute hyperopia. An eye with a small amount of hyperopia has 20/20 vision without correction at age 20 because of accommodation. At age 60, the hyperopia is unchanged in amount, but the vision without correction is 20/25 because the latent and facultative hyperopia have become _____ hyperopia.

---

360. more

---

361. Astigmatism is frequently inherited as a dominant trait.

If both parents have astigmatism (less than 50 percent/50 percent or more) of their children will probably be astigmatic.

532. accommodate

---

533. The clue to the onset of accommodation during refraction is apparent diminution in size of test characters and increase in contrast between black and white without improvement in visual acuity. Patient A notes the letters in the 20/15 line to be blacker and smaller when the minus sphere is increased above 1.00 D indicating _____ .

---

704. (1) visual requirements ⎫ either
     (2) symptoms   ⎭ order

---

705. An uncorrected myope complains of _____ .

---

876. astigmatism

---

877. The theoretical focal plane of a lens is a straight line. Deviation from the theoretical focal plane produces curvature of field. Failure of a line connecting the circles of least confusion resulting from astigmatism of oblique incidence to approximate the theoretical flat focal plane of a lens results in _____ .

17. (Your trial lens may be slightly different in shape.)

(Use a regular trial lens set for this frame.)

18. Sketch the handle of the 2.00 Spherical Convex lens.

---

189. absolute

---

190. Latent hyperopia can only be measured after relaxation of the physiologic tone of the ciliary muscles. This can be accomplished with drugs called cycloplegics which temporarily paralyze the ciliary muscles. Only in the presence of cycloplegia can the amount of _____ hyperopia be measured, in addition to absolute and facultative hyperopia, which are measurable without cycloplegics.

---

361. 50 percent or more

---

362. Large amounts of astigmatism are frequently associated with large amounts of myopia and hyperopia. When such is the case, the astigmatism follows the hereditary pattern of high myopia and hyperopia which is usually _____.

533. onset of accommodation

534. Lancaster has advised as a final check on axis of astigmatism, when using dials, that the minus cylinder **only** be removed from the final correction, allowing the conoid of Sturm to expand forward in the eye. The patient is again directed to study a 10 degree dial. When the minus cylinder is removed the anterior focal line of the recreated conoid of Sturm lies _____ to the retina and the posterior focal line lies on the retina.

705. blurred distance vision

706. Normal distance vision in healthy myopic eyes can be achieved only with full correction of the myopia. For a myopic patient who desires perfect distance vision _____ correction must be prescribed.

877. curvature of field

878. The base curve of a spherical meniscus lens is the surface with the _____ power.

18. (Your trial lens may be slightly different in shape.)

(Use a regular trial lens set for this frame.)

19. Hold the lens marked +2.00 (Spherical Convex) about 12 inches from your eye, and look through it at the edge of this frame. Move the lens slightly from side to side and note the apparent movement of the frame. What direction is this apparent movement compared to the movement of the lens?

---

190. latent

---

191. An eye with a visual acuity of 20/40 requires +0.75 D correction to obtain 20/20 vision. The absolute hyperopia measures (1) _____ D. The vision remains 20/20 with a correction of +1.25 (+1.50 gave 20/25). The facultative hyperopia measures (2) _____ D. A cycloplegic drug is instilled and 20/20 vision is obtained with +2.25 D. (Total hyperopia thus equals 2.25 D.) The latent hyperopia is (3) _____ D.

---

362. recessive

---

363. In one commonly used method of refracting an astigmatic eye, both foci must be brought in front of the retina (creating compound myopic astigmatism), the axes determined, the conoid of Sturm eliminated (reduced until both foci are together), and finally, the resultant point focus brought back to the retina.

The first step is accomplished by the use of (1) _____ spheres. This will (2) _____ the vision.

534. anterior

535. Removal of the cylinder only from the final correction of OD of patient A results in dial No. 1 appearing as in Figure 2. Figure 1 is its appearance when the eye is fogged. In this case the axis of the correcting minus cylinder is (1) _____ when the eye is fogged and (2) _____ when the posterior focal line of the conoid of Sturm is on the retina.

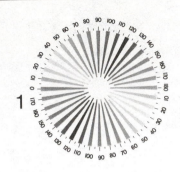 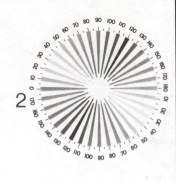

706. full (full myopic)

707. A myope without presbyopia who has a normal accommodation-convergence relationship will be comfortable reading only while his myopia is fully corrected. Many myopes do not have a normal accommodation-convergence relationship and hence will read comfortably with partial or no correction of the myopia. If a myopic patient reads comfortably without his distance correction, he may have an abnormal _____ relationship.

878. weaker (or lower)

879. The base curve of a single vision meniscus lens with a toric surface is _____ .

19. Opposite

(Use a regular trial lens set for this frame.)

20. This apparent opposite motion, which is technically termed against motion, is a common property of plus or convex lenses. Now move the same + lens up and down. What is the technical term for the direction of the apparent motion?

---

191. (1) 0.75 D
(2) 0.50 D
(3) 1.00 D

---

192. To see clearly at 14 inches (33.3 cm), the emmetropic eye must _____.

---

363. (1) plus (convex)
(2) reduce (or blur or fog)

---

364. After adding plus lenses until the vision is fogged to 20/200, we assume that both focal planes are in front of the retina. We then reduce plus by 0.25 D steps until the patient can read 20/70. If the astigmatic error is expected to be smaller than 1.00 D, the plus should be reduced until vision is improved to 20/40. If these steps are carefully done accommodation will be (relaxed/stimulated).

535. (1) 25
    (2) 25

---

536. Compare the final correction found subjectively using dials with the retinoscopic finding of OD patient A. *(Refer to Fig. 7.)* There has been a small error in determining the (sphere, and/or cylinder, and/or axis) by retinoscopy.

---

707. accommodation-convergence

---

708. Because of the variability in accommodation-convergence relationships in myopes, their use of distance glasses for near work in the absence of presbyopia and heterotropia is optional. If a myope asks whether or not he should use his glasses while reading, he will be informed their use for this purpose is _____.

---

879. the lower powered curve on the toric surface

---

880. The toric surface of a bifocal is always on the opposite surface from the segment. The base curve of a bifocal does not refer to either of the toric curves but to the curve of the surface on which the _____ is found.

20. Against motion (or against)

(Use a regular trial lens set for this frame.)

21. Hold a -2.00 (Spherical Concave) lens about 12 inches from your eye, look through it at this frame, move it from side to side slightly, and note the apparent motion of this frame. This apparent motion of the frame is (like/unlike) the apparent motion caused by the convex lens.

---

192. accommodate (accommodate 3.00 D)

---

193. Snellen letters subtend an angle of (1) _____ in height and width, with each component subtending an angle of (2) _____ at the stated distance.

---

364. relaxed

---

365. Remember that a conoid of Sturm exists for every point seen by an astigmatic eye. Thus when two lines are viewed by an astigmat who has the posterior focal line of the conoid of Sturm on the retina the line parallel with that focal line will be seen as blacker. The distance A represents the interval of Sturm. The _____ line of the cross will appear blacker to the diagrammed eye.

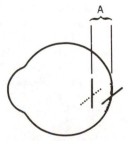

536. axis

---

537. If the retinoscopy revealed hyperopia, the entire conoid of Sturm would be moved anterior to the retina by the use of _____ spheres to pro-
(sign)
duce an artificial myopia (called fogging) for the purpose of using astigmatic dials.

---

708. optional

---

709. Hyperopes who have no absolute hyperopia require _____ correction to obtain their best distance visual acuity.

---

880. segment

---

881. Astigmatism of oblique incidence can be reduced by careful selection of base curves for various powers of lenses. When the visual axis is directed away from the optical center of a lens, astigmatism is introduced. This astigmatism can be minimized by selecting the proper _____ for the power of the lens.

21. unlike

(Use a regular trial lens set for this frame.)

22. The apparent motion caused by concave lenses is with or in the same direction as the movement of the lens. For this reason the technical term for this apparent motion caused by a concave lens is _____ motion.

---

193. (1) five minutes
     (2) one minute

---

194. If the stated distance of viewing a Snellen letter is 14 inches, the 14/14 letters will subtend an angle of (1) _____ with a separation of components of each letter of (2) _____.

---

365. horizontal

---

366. The axis of the astigmatism can be determined by placing the posterior portion of the conoid of Sturm on the retina, having the patient view radiating lines (called a clock dial) and telling us which line is blackest. If the patient sees chart A as chart B, we know then that the patient (has/has no) astigmatism.

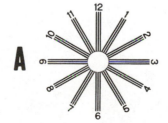 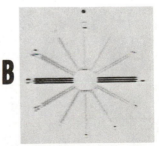

537. plus

---

538. As long as a patient is fogged, accommodation is relaxed. In this respect fogging is similar to the use of a _____.

---

709. no

---

710. The amount of facultative hyperopia to be corrected depends on the patient's symptoms. Symptoms may be negligible in the presence of considerable hyperopia if the patient does no close work. The same amount of hyperopia in a patient doing close work extensively may require full correction of facultative hyperopia. The more close work a patient does, the more likely he is to require correction of _____ hyperopia.

---

881. base curve

---

882. Spherical aberration can be minimized by the grinding of a(n) (1) _____ surface on a lens or by changing the form of the lens from a biconcave or biconvex to a (2) _____ form.

22. with

(Use a regular trial lens set for this frame.)

23. Place the $+2.00$ D lens and -2.00 D lens surface to surface. Move the pair of lenses back and forth. Note the lack of motion of an object observed through these moving lenses. This neutralized motion indicates that these two lenses are of opposite sign and of (equal/unequal) power.

---

194. (1) five minutes
     (2) one minute

---

195. In the normally accommodating eye the visual acuity at 14 inches is the same as at 20 feet. A normally accommodating emmetropic eye with a near visual acuity of 14/14 would be expected to have an acuity of _____ at 20 feet.

---

366. has

---

367. A convenient method for communicating to the patient about the direction of the lines of the clock dial is to refer to the lines as the 3-9 line or the 12-6 line.

Which line would the patient regard as the blackest in the figure?

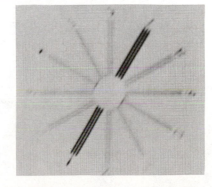

538. cycloplegic

---

539. When dials are used to subjectively test astigmatism in a hyperopic patient, it is important that the fog be maintained during the entire procedure. To assure this, as lenses are changed in the trial frame the plus sphere last in position is never removed until the next plus sphere to be used has been inserted or the patient is instructed to close his eyes while lenses are changed. If one of these procedures is not followed, the patient will be able to _____ while lenses are being changed.

---

710. facultative

---

711. Latent hyperopia can be determined only by the use of _____.

---

882. (1) aspheric
    (2) meniscus

---

883. Chromatic aberration can be reduced by using glass with a low _____ in spectacle manufacture.

23. equal

---

24. In order to understand the apparent motion properties of concave and convex lenses better, think for a moment about prisms.

Light is deflected toward the base of a prism. Object A in the diagram will appear to be located at position B. The object appears displaced toward the _____ of the prism.

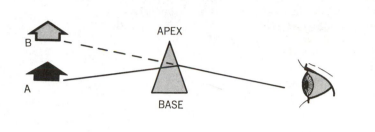

---

195. 20/20

---

196. The only standardized test of near visual acuity utilizes reduced Snellen letters at 14 inches or about 0.33 m. With this system a near visual acuity of 14/28 is equivalent to a distance visual acuity of _____.

---

367. 1-7

---

368. It is noteworthy that by picking the lower numbered hour of the two hours which describe the position of the line that the patient states is the blackest on the clock dial (as 12-6, use 6) and multiplying this by 30 you derive the minus cylinder axis. Thus, if the patient notes the 12-6 line to be the blackest, his minus cylinder axis is 6×30 or 180 degrees (and minus cylinder axis 180 degrees = with the rule astigmatism). If the patient notes the 9-3 line to be the blackest, the minus cylinder axis is (1) _____, which is (2) (with/against) the rule astigmatism.

539. accommodate

---

540. Once an astigmatic error has been neutralized with dials, the fog is slowly reduced until the best visual acuity is obtained. This is accomplished by reducing the power of the _____ sphere in the
(sign)

case of hyperopia.

---

711. cycloplegics

---

712. Because of symptoms it is sometimes necessary to correct some latent hyperopia. This results in glasses which _____ distance vision.

---

883. chromatic dispersion

---

884. Astigmatism of oblique incidence can be reduced by proper selection of _____ for a given power lens.

24. apex

(Use a regular trial lens set for this frame.)

25. Take any free prism from the trial case. Hold it away from your eyes and look through it at a horizontal object across the room. This demonstrates that the image displacement is toward the _____ of the prism.

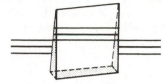

---

196. 20/40

---

197. The first test of near visual acuity was devised by an Austrian named Jaeger. The size of print of Jaeger test types (abbreviated J) has never been standardized. Despite this, near visual acuity charts for use at 14 inches frequently are calibrated in increasing size from J 1 to J 14 or more. A near visual acuity expressed as J 4 (has/has no) exact equivalent Snellen distance acuity.

---

368. (1) 90 degrees
   (2) against

---

369. We have spoken of meridians of cylinders as the line along which the greatest curvature of a cylinder lies. The term "axis" refers to the true axis of the cylinder, perpendicular to the meridian. Refraction by a cylinder results in a focal line parallel to its axis. Remember, a 90 degree axis cylinder results in a focal line at 90 degrees and a 180 degree cylinder results in a focal line at _____ .

540. plus

---

541. If retinoscopy reveals no astigmatism, its absence may be verified subjectively by fogging the patient to a visual acuity of about 20/40 and asking him to observe a fan or clock dial. If the retinoscopy has been accurate, he will note _____ lines blacker and clearer than the others.

---

712. blur (or fog)

---

713. Astigmatism with the rule is corrected by a minus cylinder near axis _____ .

---

884. base curve

---

885. Distortion of the image results from unequal magnification of points in the periphery and center of a lens. It becomes apparent only when extended objects such as an entire checkerboard are viewed.

Image distortion is an aberration due to varying _____ of points of an extended object.

25. apex

26. Two prisms, arranged as in the left diagram with reference to the eye and object A, will allow the observer to see object A in A's true position.

The two prisms are now moved down in relation to object A and the eye. Object A now appears at position B. Movement of these prisms in one direction causes the object to appear to move in the _____ direction.

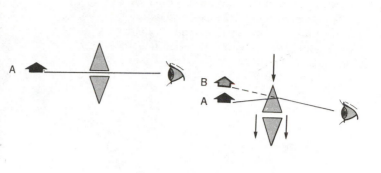

197. has no

198. Type size in printing in the United States, regardless of type style, is measured by the point system. One point is 0.35 mm or about 1/72 inch. Ten points of Fairfield Medium style print measure _____.

369. 180 degrees

370. By creating compound myopic astigmatism we have both lines of the conoid of Sturm in front of the retina, one nearer to it than the other. To move the line which is further from the retina toward the line closer to the retina (reducing the conoid of Sturm) (1) (plus/minus) (2) (spherical/cylindrical) lenses will be used.

541. no

---

542. While the maximum curvature power of a cylinder is perpendicular to the axis and its effect is always parallel to its axis, a minus cylinder at 180 degrees will create a focal line at _____ degrees.

---

713. 180 (180 degrees)

---

714. A given amount of astigmatism against the rule causes more blurring of vision, but less discomfort, than an equal amount of astigmatism with the rule. If a patient with a small amount of astigmatism complains of poor vision, it is likely to be astigmatism _____ the rule.

---

885. magnification

---

886. Distortion is of two types, barrel and pincushion. Viewing an extended object through a convex lens results in greater magnification of peripheral points than central, and its effect on a checkerboard is illustrated. Plus lenses cause _____ distortion.

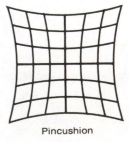

Pincushion

26. opposite

27. A plus or convex lens may be considered as two prisms placed base to base.

When object A is viewed through the center of a plus lens it is not displaced, but if the lens is moved down, the object appears displaced _____ .

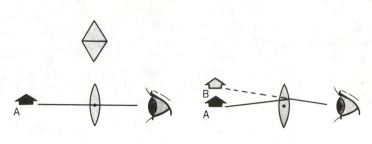

198. 3.5 mm or 10/72 inch

199. A patient is primarily interested in his ability to read customary size print. Reduced Snellen charts and Jaeger test types have no relation to the type size of ordinary literature. A system of denoting near visual acuity which is related to the print size is the point system. To express near visual acuity in relation to the size of customary reading matter, the _____ system is used.

370. (1) minus
(2) cylindrical

371. When a line stands out blacker on the clock dial, astigmatism is present. When the astigmatism has been corrected all the lines on the clock dial will appear _____ .

542. 180

---

543. A patient may fail to appreciate a difference in the lines on the astigmatic dial. To determine whether the lack of difference in lines is due to absence of astigmatism or intellectual incompetence of the patient, astigmatism may be created. Placing a minus cylinder before the fogged eye creates a conoid of Sturm, with the posterior focal line (parallel/perpendicular) to the axis of the cylinder.

---

714. against

---

715. A change in a patient's astigmatic correction which is more than about a diopter or greater than about 10 degrees is usually not well tolerated. Therefore, some compromise in prescribing new astigmatic corrections is occasionally necessary, and the full accurate correction may have to be made in steps separated by several months. Large changes in (1) _____ and (2) _____ of astigmatic corrections are occasionally not well tolerated by patients.

---

886. pincushion

---

887. Minus lenses cause greater reduction in size of peripheral points of an extended object than central, as illustrated. Concave lenses cause _____ distortion.

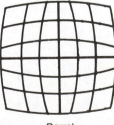

Barrel

27. up

---

28. The distance a prism bends light (prismatic power) is proportional to the angle of the apex. The greater the angle, the greater the prismatic power.

Prism A has (more/less) prismatic power than prism B.

A   B

---

199. point

---

200. Lower case letters are of three forms: ascenders, descenders, and small sorts. The lower case letter p, for example, is a descender, and d is an ascender. The lower case letters, a, r, and c, are all _____ .

---

371. the same (or equally black)

---

372. If F_2 is brought to F_1 with minus cylinder the lines of the clock dial will be _____ .

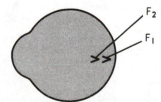

543. parallel

---

544. The line on an astigmatic dial which appears blackest is (perpendicular/parallel) to the focal line nearer the retina of a fogged eye with astigmatism.

---

715. (1) axis } either
       (2) power } order

---

716. To compromise when making large changes in cylindrical power it is useful to prescribe the spherical equivalent of the cylinder. If it is desired to cut the power of a cylinder from -3.00 D to -2.00 D, the sphere found on refraction must be altered by -0.50 D. Thus the spherical equivalent is one-half the cylinder. If you desire to reduce the cylinder from -4.00 D to -2.00 D, the sphere found on refraction must be altered by _____.

---

887. barrel

---

888. Barrel-shaped distortion occurs with (1) _____ lenses and pincushion distortion with (2) _____ lenses.

28. more

---

29. The image displacement is not constant in a spherical lens, but increases proportionately to the distance from the optical center of the lens. As the periphery of the lens is approached, greater prismatic effect is discernible.

Prismatic power at point A is _____ than prismatic power at point B.

---

200. small sorts

---

201. Clues to the perception of a word are provided by ascenders and descenders. Near vision test types based on the point system utilize only small sorts to eliminate perceptual clues. The word, paper, (is/is not) a good word to use for near visual acuity testing.

---

372. the same (or equally black)

---

373. After determining the axis with the clock dial, switch to Lancaster dial No. 2 which is a chart with a movable disc with two lines perpendicular to each other. This dial is set so one of the lines corresponds to the axis already determined on the clock dial. Then minus cylinders are added in 0.25 D steps until the lines are equally black. When both lines are equal the conoid of Sturm has been _____.

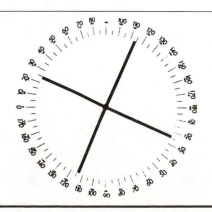

544. parallel

---

545. A patient's awareness of blacker lines on an astigmatic dial may be tested by creating astigmatism. This may be done by placing a minus cylinder before a fogged eye. Under these circumstances the patient should report that some lines are blacker. The blacker lines will be (parallel/perpendicular) to the axis at which you have placed the minus cylinder.

---

716. −1.00 D

---

717. No compromise in axis is feasible. The cylinder should always be prescribed on axis even if markedly different from the patient's previous prescription. The alternatives to prescribing the exact cylindrical findings are to prescribe no cylinder or

_____ .

---

888. (1) minus
(2) plus

---

889. Distortion is greater through flat lenses than curved. Selection of a curved form of lens will tend to diminish _____ .

29. less

(Use a regular trial lens set for this frame.)

30. We have seen that spherical power shows either with or against motion with movement of the lens. Look through any free prism and note the image displacement; now move the prism side to side and up and down. The displacement of the image is constant. The lack of relative movement of the displaced image indicates that the prism has no spherical _____.

---

201. is not

---

202. Near visual acuity is tested at a distance of _____ from the eye.

---

373. eliminated

---

374. If we are using minus cylinders to move F_2 back toward F_1 and we want the patient to remain fogged or artificially myopic (too much plus), we must add plus spheres as F_2 approaches F_1 lest the focal planes be too close to or straddle the retina. A useful rule is to add a $+0.25$ D sphere for every -0.50 D cylinder necessary to eliminate the astigmatism.

What is the desired position of F_1 and F_2, in relation to the retina, after the cylindrical correction has been determined and the eye is still fogged?

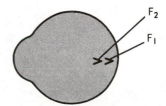

545. parallel

---

546. The spherical equivalent is that lens which places the circle of least confusion on the retina. The spherical equivalent is the total of the spherical ametropia plus one-half the cylinder. For example if the correcting lens were $+3.25 - 1.50 \times 180$ then the spherical equivalent would be $+2.50$ D sphere. If the correcting lens were $+4.50 - 1.00 \times 90$, the spherical equivalent would be _____.

---

717. cut the power of the cylinder

---

718. Asthenopia is the clinical condition of nonspecific ocular discomfort attributed to refractive errors. Asthenopic symptoms include burning, pulling, tearing, tiredness of the eyes, and, rarely, headache. A nonspecific term referring to ocular discomfort attributed to refractive error is _____.

---

889. distortion

---

890. Draw a meniscus lens.

30. power

---

31. Plus (convex) lenses positioned with the optical center below the visual axis, as diagrammed, will exert a prismatic effect. This prismatic effect is that of placing a prism with its base _____ in front of the eye.

Visual axis — Optical center — Fovea

---

202. 14 inches (0.33 m approximately)

---

203. There are three generally used methods of measuring visual acuity at near: reduced Snellen characters at 14 inches, Jaeger test types, and _____ .

---

374. In front of the retina (F_1 and F_2 coincide)

---

375. Having determined the power and axis of the cylinder, while keeping the eye myopic, we now reduce the _____ until the point focus created by elimination of the astigmatism is moved back to the retina and the eye achieves its best corrected visual acuity.

546. +4.00 D

---

547. What are the spherical equivalents of the following?

$$+5.00 - 2.50 \times 90 \ (1) \ \underline{\hspace{3cm}}.$$
$$-4.00 - 1.50 \times 90 \ (2) \ \underline{\hspace{3cm}}.$$

---

718. asthenopia

---

719. Because of the nonspecific nature of asthenopic symptoms, it is sometimes difficult to be sure that a given refractive error is indeed responsible for symptoms. The concept of what constitutes a significant refractive error thus becomes a matter of individual interpretation based on experience. It is safe to say that errors in judgment more often lead to correction of insignificant errors than noncorrection of significant errors. Should every refractive error be corrected?

890.

---

891. Lenses which are designed to minimize aberrations are known as corrected curve or best form lenses. Most modern spectacle lenses are of this type, namely, meniscus lenses with base curves varied depending upon the power of the lens. The modern meniscus lenses with base curves varied for different powers are known as _____ lenses.

31. down

---

32. Prisms arranged apex to apex, but separated, allow the object to be viewed in its usual position, A.

Movement of these prisms down causes the object A to appear to move to position B, causing apparent motion in the _____ direction as the prisms are moved.

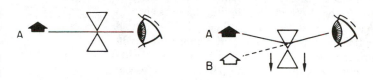

---

203. the point system (or point type)

---

204. The three generally used methods of measuring near visual acuity are (1) _____, (2) _____ and (3) _____.

---

375. spherical plus (or fog or myopia)

---

376. Since both eyes of a patient are seldom the same, it is imperative that each eye be tested separately. The axis of the astigmatism is often related between the two eyes. Frequently the cylindrical axes of the two eyes, when added together, will equal 180 degrees.

If one eye is $-C \times 80$ degrees there is a fair chance that the other eye will be $-C \times$ _____.

547. (1) +3.75 D
(2) −4.75 D

548. In hyperopic astigmatism, large astigmatic errors may produce so much blur of vision that pinpointing of blacker lines on a fan type astigmatic dial is difficult. To improve the accuracy of dials in this type of case it may be necessary to move the posterior focal line of the conoid of Sturm behind the retina. Accommodation will be relaxed provided the circle of least confusion remains well anterior to the retina. The spherical lens which will produce this position of the conoid within the eye will be (more/less) convex than the spherical equivalent.

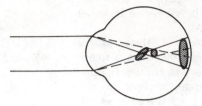

Fogged Hyperopic High Astigmatism

719. No

720. We have emphasized the important relationship between accommodation and the refractive state. It is also apparent that responses on subjective testing may be variable in accuracy. For these reasons refractions cannot be as precise as measurement of lenses on a lensometer; nevertheless, results of refraction are surprisingly reproducible within small margins of error. Is refraction mathematically precise?

891. corrected curve (or best form)

892. The general terms used to describe lenses which minimize aberrations are (1) _____
and (2) _____.

32. same

---

33. The object at position A would appear in its true position if viewed through the center of a minus lens and between the apices of two prisms. If the prisms or the minus lens are moved down, the object will appear to move _____ .

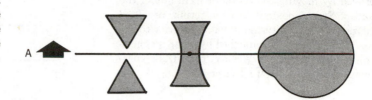

---

204. (1) Jaeger test types } in
   (2) reduced Snellen characters for use at 14 inches } any
   (3) point system } order

205. Six point type when read at 14 inches is approximately equivalent to 14/28. Six point type is used in telephone directories. A patient normally accommodating who has no difficulty reading the telephone directory at 14 inches could be expected to have a corrected distance acuity of _____ or better.

---

376. 100 degrees

---

377. A conoid of Sturm may be produced to verify the axis and power of the astigmatic correction. This is done with a **cross cylinder**. This lens is composed of either 0.12, 0.25, 0.37, 0.50, or 1.00 D cylinders in this fashion:

$$+0.25 \times 180 \bigcirc -0.25 \times 90.$$

This lens would have $+0.25$ D power in the 90 degree meridian and _____ in the 180 degree meridian.

548. more

---

549. Similarly in myopic astigmatism of high degree, accuracy of fan type astigmatic dials may be improved by moving the posterior focal line of the conoid of Sturm posterior to the retina, provided the circle of least confusion remains anterior to the retina. This can be accomplished by using a spherical minus lens (stronger/weaker) than the spherical equivalent of the refractive error.

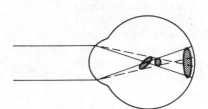

Fogged Hyperopic High Astigmatism

---

720. No

---

721. The margins of error of refraction techniques in spherical and cylindrical power approach ± 0.25 D. A hyperope may be uncomfortable if overcorrected 0.25 D for distance, and a myope may suffer reduction of visual acuity of one line if undercorrected 0.25 D. Generally, however, changes in spherical and cylindrical power of 0.25 D are within the _____ of refraction techniques.

---

892. (1) corrected curve ⎫ either
      (2) best form   ⎭ order

---

893. As a result of chromatic aberration within the eye, red rays are refracted less than green. If the focal point of a spot of white light is on the retina, there will thus be a green focal point slightly in front of the retina and a red focal point slightly behind. If an eye is hyperopic and uncorrected by neither accommodation nor plus lenses, parallel green rays will be focused (closer to/farther from) the retina than parallel red rays.

33. down

---

34. Minus (concave) lenses positioned with the optical center above the visual axis will exert a prismatic effect. This prismatic effect on the visual axis is that of placing a prism base _____ in front of the eye.

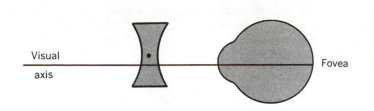

Visual axis

Fovea

---

205. 20/40

---

206. A near vision test chart which provides acuity values in all three methods is the Lebensohn chart. Twelve point type is approximately equivalent to what distance visual acuity and is found in what type of reading material? *(See Figs. 5 and 6, pp. 351, 352.)*

---

377. -0.25 D

---

378. A 0.25 D cross cylinder is written: $+0.25 \times 180 \bigcirc -0.25 \times 90$.

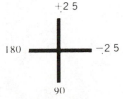

In plus cylinder form this is written: _____.

549. weaker

---

550. Retinoscopy may be subjectively verified by a technique utilizing astigmatic dials or by using cross cylinders. Astigmatic dials and cross cylinder techniques are methods of _____ the findings of retinoscopy.

---

721. margins of error

---

722. A patient is wearing $+3.75 - 2.00 \times 135$ OU. Your refraction shows $+4.00 - 2.25 \times 135$ OU. Is it usually necessary to change these lenses?

---

893. closer to

---

894. Chromatic aberration occurring within the eye is the basis of a clinical test in refraction known as the duochrome test. The patient is asked to compare the clarity of test characters printed on a red background with the clarity of equal size characters on a green background. If the refraction has been precise, the characters will be equally clear on the red and green backgrounds. In the duochrome test, the end point is _____.

34. down

---

35. You have learned that *against motion* occurs with plus lenses. There is one exception to this rule. If the object viewed and the observer are both farther from a plus lens than the focal distance, *with motion* occurs. If the observer is within the focal distance of a plus lens _____ motion of the image occurs.

---

206. 20/80. Books of children age 9–12

---

207. In different styles of printing, the relationship between the length of ascenders and descenders and the height of small sorts varies. The Lebensohn chart used Century Schoolbook type in which small sorts are one-half the designated point size. On the Lebensohn chart a 10 point (1 point = 0.35 mm) small sort is _____ mm high.

---

378. $-0.25 + 0.50 \times 180$

---

379. The magnitude of the conoid of Sturm is indicated by the power of the cylinder of a spherocylindrical combination. A 0.25 D cross cylinder ($+0.25 - 0.50 \times 90$) has a conoid of Sturm of 0.50 D. How large is the conoid of Sturm of a 0.50 D cross cylinder (in diopters)?

550. verifying

---

551. When cross cylinders are to be used to verify retinoscopy, the net or corrected finding is first placed in the trial frame. On the basis of the retinoscopy, patient A's lenses OS to be verified, and hence to be placed in the trial frame, are _____. *(Refer to data sheet; see Fig. 7.)*

---

722. No

---

723. The margins of error of refraction techniques in spherical and cylindrical powers are _____.

---

894. equal clarity of letters on the red and green backgrounds

---

895. A test for determining when the focal plane of entering rays is on the retina, based on chromatic aberration within the eye, is known as the _____ test.

35. against

(Use a regular trial lens set for this frame.)

36. The focal distance of a +5.00 D lens is 8 inches. When this lens is held farther away from the eye than 8 inches and objects at 20 feet or more are viewed, the image is (upright/inverted).

(Perform and observe this with a +5.00 D lens.)

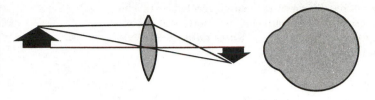

---

207. 1.75 mm or 5/72 inch
($\frac{1}{2}$ of 3.5 mm or $\frac{1}{2}$ of 10/72 inch)

---

208. When a patient's near visual acuity is being tested he should be wearing his near correction to minimize any deficiency of accommodation and refractive error. Tests of near vision are made with the patient wearing his _____.

---

379. 1.00 D

---

380. A 0.75 D cross cylinder is composed of

$$+0.75 \times 180 \bigcirc -0.75 \times 90, \text{ or}$$
$$+0.75 - 1.50 \times 90$$

Of what magnitude (in diopters) is the conoid of Sturm created by a 0.75 D cross cylinder?

551. $-1.00 - 1.50 \times 180$

552. Accuracy using cross cylinders requires that the circle of least confusion (or point focus, if cylinder has corrected all of the astigmatism) be on the retina. This position can be verified by moving the circle of least confusion anteriorly and posteriorly with _____ lenses until the best visual acuity is obtained.

723. ± 0.25 D

724. An exception to the rule of not changing spherical power less than 0.50 D occurs in the case of advanced presbyopes who frequently will appreciate a 0.25 D change in add. When the amplitude of accommodation is markedly restricted, near correction may be increased as little as _____ D with relief of the patient's symptoms.

895. duochrome

896. A patient with uncorrected myopia will see test characters more clearly against the _____ background in the duochrome test.

36. inverted

---

37. When inverted images of distant objects are viewed through a plus lens which is held farther from the eye than the focal distance, moving the lens down causes an unusual motion for a plus lens. Such a downward movement causes a prism base down effect but shows a(n) _____ motion.

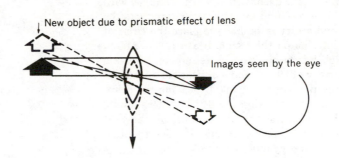

New object due to prismatic effect of lens

Images seen by the eye

---

208. near correction

---

209. Legal forms occasionally ask for monocular recording of near visual acuity, but for practical purposes, in the absence of significant visual loss due to disease, it is generally tested binocularly. If a patient's vision can be corrected to 20/20 in each eye it is the general practice to measure his near visual acuity (binocularly/monocularly).

---

380. 1.50 D

---

381. A cross cylinder has a handle so oriented that the lens may be conveniently rotated by a simple twist of the handle to reverse the position of the plus and minus axes. In the photograph the plus cylinder axis is parallel to 135 degrees; if the handle is twisted, turning the lens over, then the _____ cylinder axis is parallel to 135 degrees.

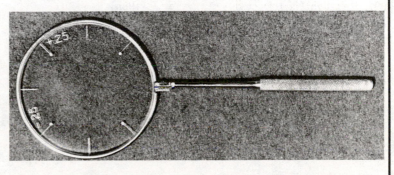

552. spherical

---

553. The spherical lens which, when combined with the cylinder as found by retinoscopy, produces the best visual acuity is assumed to place the circle of least confusion on the retina. If a $+1.00 \; -2.00 \times 90$, which has been found by retinoscopy, gives a visual acuity of 20/50, and substitutions of various spheres in place of the $+1.00$ D (leaving the cylinder the same) shows that a $+0.25$ D sphere results in the best visual acuity of 20/30, then the working lenses to be placed before this eye in preparation for cross cylinder verification are _____.

---

724. 0.25

---

725. The greater the power of the cylinder, the more precisely the axis of cylinder can be refined. It is difficult in most cases to accurately place a 0.25 D cylinder, and the margins of error of axis determination of a 0.50 D cylinder are 5 to 10 degrees in either direction. A patient is wearing $+2.50 - 0.50 \times 170$. Your refraction shows $+2.50 - 0.50 \times 175$. Is it usually necessary to change this lens?

---

896. red

---

897. Red light is refracted _____ than green in the eye.

37. with

(Use a regular trial lens set for this frame.)

38. Base down prism effect of the downward displacement of the plus lens displaces the object up. Since all images are inverted, this results in the image being displaced farther down and giving a(n) _____ motion when a plus lens is moved down while being held outside the focal distance of the lens. Hold a +5.00 D (spherical convex) lens at arm's length and observe the apparent motion as an object across the room is observed while the lens is moved.

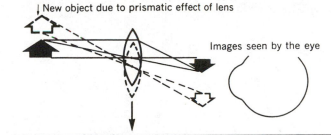

New object due to prismatic effect of lens

Images seen by the eye

---

209. binocularly

---

210. The amplitude of accommodation is greater when tested binocularly than monocularly. A patient with 6.00 D of accommodation in the right eye can be expected to have (1) _____ D in the left eye and (2) (more than/less than) 6.00 D when both eyes are tested simultaneously.

---

381. minus

---

382. The handle of the cross cylinder is 45 degrees from each axis of the cross cylinder. The diagram shows straddling of a 90 degree cylinder axis by a cross cylinder. To straddle an axis with the cross cylinder, place the handle of the cross cylinder _____ to the proposed axis.

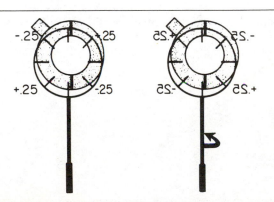

553. $+0.25 - 2.00 \times 90$

---

554. When cross cylinders are used to verify the axis and power of astigmatism, the eye being tested (is/is not) fogged.

---

725. No

---

726. The necessity of prescribing a small correction or a small change in correction is governed not only by the margins of error of refraction techniques but also by the limitations of the optician in grinding lenses and the placement of spectacles on the patient's face.

Accuracy in refraction, accuracy in filling the prescription, and accuracy in _____ on the patient are all subject to small unavoidable errors.

---

897. less

---

898. Prism power through the optical center of a lens is _____.

38. with

---

39. Prismatic power is usually noted in prism diopters. One prism diopter is that amount of power which will deviate parallel light 1 cm when measured 1 m behind the lens.

A prism with a power of 2 prism diopters will deviate parallel rays of light _____ cm when measured 1 m behind the prism.

---

210. (1) 6
(2) more than

---

211. The amplitude of accommodation is greater when tested binocularly than when each eye is tested separately. With the distance correction in place, the binocular near point can be expected to be _____ than the monocular near point.

---

382. parallel

---

383. Cross cylinders are used to verify the axis and power of proposed cylindrical corrections. There are several ways of establishing a tentative cylindrical correction. A means of verifying astigmatic correction is by use of the _____ .

554. is not

---

555. Cross cylinders will be used to verify the retinoscopy of patient A. OD is occluded and -1.00 -1.50×180 is put in the trial frame before OS. The visual acuity with this combination of lenses is $20/25 - 3$. Trial of $-1.25 - 1.50 \times 180$ gave no improvement and $-0.75 - 1.50 \times 180$ resulted in a vision of $20/30$. The lenses to be used as working lenses for the cross cylinder verification are _____. *(Record the visual acuity obtained with this combination on the data sheet; see Fig. 7.)*

---

726. placement of spectacles
(or equivalent words)

---

727. The higher the power of a cylinder, the lower the tolerance of error of axis placement by the optician. Will an axis placement error of a 4.00 D cylinder be tolerated as well as the same error of placement of a 0.50 D cylinder?

---

898. zero

---

899. All spectacle lenses produce prismatic power as gaze is shifted from the optical center of a lens. If the correction is roughly equal in each eye, the prismatic power will be _____ in each eye for each direction of gaze.

39. 2

---

40. An ophthalmic lens is said to be decentered when its optical center is not aligned with the visual axis. When a 1 D lens (+ or −) is decentered 1 cm from the visual axis, there will be 1 *prism diopter* deviation.

When a 4 D lens (+ or −) is decentered 1 cm from the visual axis, there will be a 4 *prism diopters* deviation. From this we can say that

Prism diopters = decentration (in cm) × _____.

---

211. nearer (or closer)

---

212. A patient who has difficulty following a line of print to the right but no difficulty beginning a sentence may have a _____ .

---

383. cross cylinder

---

384. To verify a proposed cylindrical axis the handle of the cross cylinder is held parallel with this proposed axis thus "straddling" it. Keeping the handle in the same axis it is turned so that the cross cylinder lens flips over, exchanging the minus cross cylinder axis with the plus cross cylinder axis.

To verify a proposed cylindrical axis the handle is held _____ to the proposed axis.

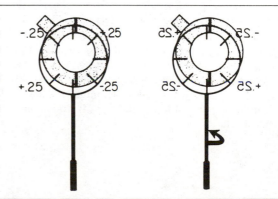

555. $-1.00 - 1.50 \times 180$ *(Record on data sheet; see Fig. 7.)*

556. The total cylindrical power of a $+0.50 \times 180$ ⌒ -0.50×90 cross cylinder is _____ .

727. No

728. Despite the accuracy of determination and placement of the axis of a large cylinder, one factor beyond the control of refractionist and optician is the change in position of the frame after the patient obtains his spectacles. Variation in axis of cylinders occurs after the patient obtains his spectacles due to changes in _____ .

899. equal

900. A patient wearing a $+1.00$ OD and -1.00 OS has 0.8Δ base (1) _____ OD and 0.8Δ base (2) _____ OS while looking through the lenses 8 mm below the optical centers. The above lenses create a vertical phoria which will total (3) _____ Δ while looking through this point. The induced vertical imbalance is a (4) (right/left) hyperphoria.

40. power (in diopters)

---

41. Decentering a plus lens up results in base (1) _____ prism in the visual axis, while decentering a minus lens up results in base (2) _____ prism in the visual axis.

+Lens

−Lens

---

212. right (homonymous) hemianopsia

---

213. A patient who, on reaching the right edge of a line of print which he has read correctly, has difficulty locating the beginning of the next line may have a _____ .

---

384. parallel

---

385. A new cylinder at a slightly different axis is effectively created when the cross cylinder straddles a proposed axis. The new cylinder's axis is changed by an equal number of degrees in the opposite direction by flipping the cross cylinder. When the handle is flipped while parallel to the proposed axis, two new cylinders are created each of which is a(n) _____ number of degrees from the proposed axis.

556. 1.00 D

---

557. If retinoscopy is thought to have been reasonably accurate, the lower the power of the cross cylinder used the more sensitive the test. In no event should the total cylindrical power of the cross cylinder exceed the presumed power of the cylinder. A $+1.00$ C $\times$ 180 $\subset$ -1.00 C $\times$ 90 for cross cylinder (is/is not) suitable for verifying the astigmatism of $\overline{OS}$, patient A as determined by retinoscopy. *(Refer to data sheet; see Fig. 7.)*

---

728. positions of the frame

---

729. Because of the several reasons extended, it is generally acceptable to prescribe the axis of cylinders to the nearest multiple of 5 degrees with the possible exception of very high power cylinders such as 4.00 D or more. Your refraction shows $+2.00 - 1.00 \times 173$. It is acceptable to prescribe $+2.00 - 1.00 \times$ _____ .

---

900. (1) up   (3) 1.6
(2) down   (4) right

---

901. The power used in the formula Prism diopters = power $\times$ decentration will be different in various meridians if a cylinder is present. In calculating the prismatic effect anywhere along the vertical meridian of a $+6.00 -1.00 \times 180$ lens, the power used is 5.00 D (-1.00 D cylinder at axis 180 results in $+5.00$ D curve in the vertical meridian of this lens.) Hence, 10 mm above the optical center the prismatic power will be (1) _____ Δ base (2) _____ .

41. (1) up
(2) down

---

42. Prism diopters = decentration (cm) × power (D).

If a 10.00 D lens is decentered 1 mm (0.1 cm), the prismatic effect will be _____ prism diopter(s).

---

213. left (homonymous) hemianopsia

---

214. Myopia is the refractive state of too much plus in the eye for distant vision. An uncorrected 3.00 D myopic eye requires about _____
D of accommodation to read the 14/14 line on the near chart held at 0.33 m.

---

385. equal

---

386. To verify a proposed axis using the cross cylinder, the patient is asked which position of the cross cylinder when it is flipped (handle parallel to proposed axis) provides clearer vision. If vision is equally blurred in both positions the proposed axis is correct.

If on flipping the cross cylinder, the proposed axis is correct the patient will report _____ .

557. is not

---

558. The 0.25 D cross cylinder ($+0.25 \times 180$ -0.25×90) is used more frequently than the other cross cylinders. The 0.25 D cross cylinder has a total cylindrical power of _____ .

---

729. 175

---

730. Since the symptoms produced by heterophorias are often indistinguishable from asthenopia due to refractive errors, it is often difficult to decide whether or not to prescribe treatment for the heterophoria. Symptoms caused by heterophoria resemble _____ .

---

901. (1) 5
(2) down

---

902. If the meridian of a lens under consideration is parallel to the cylinder axis, then the cylindrical power need not be considered when calculating prismatic effect in that meridian. A $+6.00 -1.00$ $\times 90$ lens has (1) _____ Δ base (2) _____ at a point 10 mm superior to the optical center.

42. 1

---

43. Prism diopter is abbreviated Δ.

Using the formula, Δ = decentration (cm) × power (D), when a +5.00 D lens is decentered down 4 mm, the prismatic effect will be (1) _____ Δ base (2) _____.

---

214. zero

---

215. Hyperopia is the refractive state of too little plus in the eye. An uncorrected 5.00 D hyperopic eye requires 5.00 D accommodation for clear distant vision and will require a total of _____ D accommodation for clear vision at 0.33 m.

---

386. equally blurred vision in both positions (or equivalent words)

---

387. If, in verifying an axis using a cross cylinder, the patient reports one position provides clearer vision than the other position, the axis is not correct. The proposed axis is changed by rotating it toward the position of the cross cylinder axis with the same sign as the correcting cylinder while the cross cylinder is in the position which provides clearer vision; i.e., if minus cylinders are used, rotate the cylinder toward the minus axis of the cross cylinder (cross cylinder in clearer position). The illustration utilizes a minus cylinder. Indicate the direction of rotation of the minus cylinder in the diagrammed circumstances. The top sequence is an example.

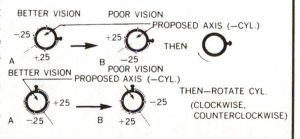

558. 0.50 D

---

559. A cross cylinder creates a conoid of Sturm with the circle of least confusion remaining coincident with the focus prior to the placement of the cross cylinder; thus cross cylinders have a net spherical power or spherical equivalent power of

_____.

---

730. asthenopia (due to refractive errors)

---

731. If both a significant refractive error and heterophoria are present, it is usually advisable to first correct the refractive error and then reevaluate the symptoms after the patient has been wearing his correction for several weeks. A patient complaining of asthenopia is found to have a significant refractive error in each eye and 6Δ esophoria. The first approach to treating this patient will be to prescribe a correction for his _____.

---

902. (1) 6
(2) down

---

903. If a patient is wearing OD $+3.00 -2.00 \times 180$ and OS $+2.00 -1.00 \times 90$, 9 mm below the optical center there is (1) _____ Δ base (2) _____ OD and (3) _____ Δ base (4) _____ OS.

43. (1) 2
   (2) down

---

44. Δ = decentration (cm) $\times$ power (D).

The prismatic effect of a -10.00 D lens decentered up 2 mm above the visual axis will be (1) _____ Δ base (2) _____ .

---

215. 8.00

---

216. At age 40 the average amplitude of accommodation is _____ .

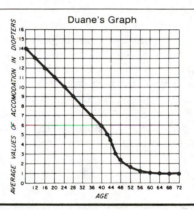

---

387. Clockwise

---

388. To refine the axis of a proposed minus cylinder it is usually best to move it in five degree steps until the patient reports equal vision in both positions.

In the diagram the proposed minus cylinder will be moved (1) _____ degrees in (2) _____ direction.

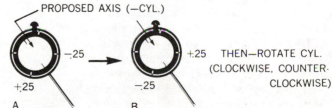

POOR VISION   BETTER VISION

PROPOSED AXIS (−CYL.)

−.25 → +.25   THEN—ROTATE CYL.
                (CLOCKWISE, COUNTER-
+.25   −.25   CLOCKWISE)

A   B

559. zero (or plano)

---

560. When cross cylinders are used, the axis of astigmatism is verified prior to the power. The cross cylinder will thus first be held before the eye with an axis (parallel to/45 degrees away from) the presumed axis of astigmatism.

---

731. refractive error

---

732. If, in your opinion, some correction for a heterophoria is indicated, vertical prisms may be considered for a vertical phoria. In the case of a large esophoria at near and an abnormal ACA ratio, plus spheres for near might be considered even in the absence of a refractive error. A patient has 12Δ E′ and an ACA ratio of 6/1 with no refractive error. You will prescribe (plus spheres/ prisms) for use at near.

---

903. (1) 0.9   (3) 1.8
(2) up   (4) up

---

904. Prismatic effects of lenses are generally not a cause of symptoms in glasses which are used exclusively for distance, provided the optical centers are aligned with the visual axes. Lateral and vertical direction of gaze are not sustained for significant periods. Distance glasses which are also used for reading may give difficulty in the reading position because of convergence at near and a tendency to look below the geometrical centers of the lenses. Symptoms due to prismatic effects of an anisometropic correction are not expected from spectacles used for _____ exclusively.

44. (1) 2

(2) down

---

45. The formula for calculating the prismatic effect of decentration of lenses is:

Prism diopters = _____ .

---

216. 6.00 D

---

217. Comfort doing near work at any given distance requires that about 50 percent of available accommodation be kept in reserve, or to state it another way, the amplitude of accommodation should be twice the accommodation required at a given distance. In order to read comfortably at 14 inches (0.33 m), an eye with no refractive error should have an accommodative amplitude of at least _____ D (approximately).

---

388. (1) 5

(2) clockwise

---

389. After verifying the axis a proposed cylindrical power can be verified with a cross cylinder. The diagram illustrates the power verifying procedure.

If better vision is reported with additional minus of the cross cylinder, give (more/less) minus cylindrical power.

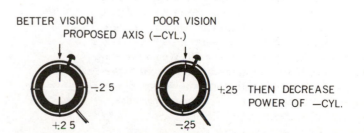

BETTER VISION   POOR VISION
PROPOSED AXIS (−CYL.)

−.25   +.25 THEN DECREASE POWER OF −CYL.

+.25   −.25

560. 45 degrees away from

---

561. In order to accurately compare the effect of various lenses on the clarity of test characters, the patient must be directed to study only characters which he can see without difficulty. A useful rule is to ask him to observe the lowest or next to lowest line of the Snellen chart which he can read without a single error with the working lenses in position. In the case of OS of patient A which line, (20/30, 20/25), will be regarded by the patient during cross cylinder testing? *(Refer to data sheet; see Fig. 7.)*

---

732. plus spheres

---

733. Symptoms due to horizontal heterophorias are not eliminated by prisms. A patient with symptoms attributed to 15Δ exophoria (may/may not) be relieved by prescription of base in prisms.

---

904. distance

---

905. If the difference in vertical prism power is 1Δ or less, there is usually no production of symptoms. Induced hyperphoria of greater than 1Δ may produce symptoms. A patient wears OD +3.00 −1.00 × 180 and OS +1.00 −1.00 × 90. Would you expect him to have symptoms due to induced hyperphoria while looking through the lenses 8 mm below the optical centers for prolonged periods?

45. decentration (cm) × power (D)

---

46. A *with motion* can be produced if a plus lens is held away from the eye more than the focal distance and the object viewed is also farther than the focal distance. To avoid this, lenses should be neutralized by holding them _____ to the eye, thus remaining within the focal distance.

---

217. 6.00

---

218. When, because of the normal decrease of accommodation with age, an individual becomes inconvenienced by blur or discomfort while performing his usual tasks at near, the condition known as presbyopia has developed. The term describing the clinical condition of lack of adequate accommodative amplitude for near work is _____.

---

389. more

---

390. To verify the power of a proposed cylinder, if the patient reports better vision when the plus axis of the cross cylinder parallels the minus cylinder axis (as diagrammed). You would give (more/less) minus power.

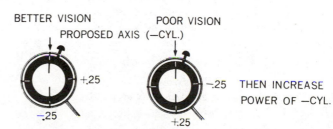

561. 20/30

562. While patient A is looking at the 20/30 line of the Snellen chart ($-1.00 - 1.50 \times 180$ in the trial frame), the 0.25 D cross cylinder is held with the axes 45 degrees to the presumed axis of the astigmatism. When the minus axis of the cross cylinder is toward 135 degrees (position 1) the numbers appear as in Figure 1; and when the minus axis is toward 45 degrees (position 2) the numbers appear as in Figure 2. The patient will reply to your questioning that the numbers are clearer when the cross cylinder is in position _____ .

E D F C Z P 30 FT. / 9.14 M **6**

1

E D F C Z P 20 FT. / 6.10 M **6**

2

---

733. may not

734. The effect of vertical prisms you intend to prescribe may be assessed by asking the patient to note any change in clarity of distance or near test characters when the prisms are held before his binocular correction. If no effect is noted, you may be reasonably certain that prisms will not be beneficial. If the clarity of test characters improves when vertical prisms are held before his correction the prisms probably (will/will not) be indicated.

---

905. No

906. Net binocular prismatic effect of lenses is the sum of the prismatic effect in each eye if the base is in before each eye and the sum if the base is out before each eye.

$$OD = 2\Delta \text{ base in} \qquad OS = 3\Delta \text{ base in}$$
$$OU = 5\Delta \text{ base in}$$

But if $OD = 4\Delta$ base in and $OS = 5\Delta$ base out, then OU = (1) _____ base (2) _____ .

46. close

---

47. The sign of an unknown lens can be found by noting the direction of the apparent motion of an image it produces. With motion implies a _____
(sign)
lens.

---

218. presbyopia

---

219. For comfort doing near work at a given distance _____ percent of the accommodation should be in reserve.

---

390. less

---

391. The axis of the astigmatism has been verified. When the minus cross cylinder axis is parallel with a -2.00 cylinder axis 180 degrees before the eye, the patient reports vision is clearer than when the plus cross cylinder axis is parallel with 180 degrees. We infer from this that more minus cylinders are needed to shorten the patient's conoid of Sturm and we add minus cylinder axis _____.

562. 1

---

563. The presumed axis of astigmatism is 180 degrees and the patient sees the characters clearer when the minus cylinder axis of the cross cylinder is along 135 degrees than when it is along 45 degrees. The minus cylinder in the trial frame should be rotated toward axis _____.

---

734. will

---

735. Prism power may easily, but expensively, be ground onto spectacle lenses. Unless absolute certainty as to their value exists, it is advisable to prescribe prisms in a frame which may be clipped onto spectacles for trial. If clip-on prisms alleviate symptoms, prism power may then be _____ spectacle lenses.

---

906. (1) 1Δ
     (2) out

---

907. A patient wears OD + 3.00 − 4.00 × 90 and OS + 3.00 − 2.00 × 90. He reads with each eye 2 mm nasal to the optical centers of his spectacles. The prismatic effect in reading is OD (1) _____ Δ base (2) _____ and OS (3) _____ Δ base (4) _____ . The net binocular prismatic effect is (5) _____ Δ.

47.  −

---

48. The power of a lens of opposite sign which neutralizes the apparent motion is a measure of the power of an unknown lens. A −4.00 D lens neutralizes the against motion of a _____ D lens.

(sign and power)

---

219. 50

---

220. After what age can presbyopia be expected to appear in the average emmetropic patient working at 14 inches? _____. Remember the patient must keep 50 percent of his accommodation in reserve.

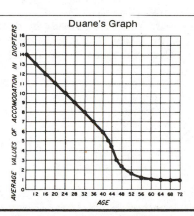

Duane's Graph

---

391. 180 degrees

---

392. When refining power using the cross cylinder, it is usually best to change the cylinder in 0.25 D steps until equal vision with both positions of the cross cylinder is reported. If the patient reports better vision with the minus cross cylinder axis at 180 degrees and the proposed cylinder is −2.00 × 180 degrees the next cylinder to be tried will be (1) _____ D × (2) _____.

563. 135 degrees

---

564. In verifying the axis of astigmatism with cross cylinders, the axis of the cylinder in the trial frame is rotated in steps of 5 degrees until the patient responds that characters have the same clarity with the cross cylinder in either position. This response indicates that the axis of the cylinder in the trial frame is (correct/incorrect).

---

735. ground onto (or incorporated in)

---

736. Prism power, when prescribed, is divided equally between the lenses. If 4Δ is to be prescribed for a patient, the prescription for each lens will include _____.

---

907. (1) 0.2   (4) out
      (2) in   (5) zero
      (3) 0.2

---

908. If prismatic effect due to spectacles is expected in a given position of gaze, this may be compensated by decentering the optical centers of the lenses with reference to the position of the visual axes during distance looking. Conversely, if prismatic effect is to be avoided, careful attention to centering the optical centers is indicated. Management of expected prismatic effect of spectacles is by _____ the optical centers of the lenses.

48. + 4.00

(Use a regular trial lens for this frame.)

49. Neutralize a − 5.00 D spherical lens from the trial case with the appropriate lens. The appropriate lens is (1) _____ and is of (2) _____ sign.

---

220. 40

221. An uncorrected hyperope of 3.00 D will be able to read comfortably at 14 inches until age _____. (3.00 D for hyperopia + 3.00 D for 0.33 m = 6.00 D required, plus an equal amount of accommodation held in reserve for comfort.)

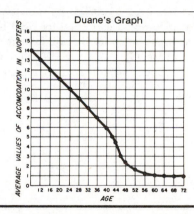

Duane's Graph

---

392. (1) − 2.25
(2) 180 degrees

393. The end point of the astigmatic power test, utilizing a cross cylinder, occurs when the patient states that both positions are equally blurred.

If the patient reports vision to be clearer when the plus cylinder axis of the cross cylinder is parallel to the minus cylinder before the eye, you must _____ the minus cylinder.

564. correct (the same as the axis of astigmatism)

565. When the cylinder before OS of patient A was rotated to 175 degrees, response to cross cylinder verification of axis was the same as in frame 562. The cylinder is now rotated to axis 170 degrees and this axis is tested with the 0.25 D cross cylinder. As the cross cylinder is flipped while holding the handle parallel to 170 degrees the patient reports the letters are equally blurred in both positions. What is the correct axis of astigmatism?

736. 2Δ

737. A patient requires 3Δ correction for right hyperphoria. The prescription for OD will include (1) _____ base (2) _____ and for OS (3) _____ base (4) _____.

908. decentering

909. Because of the prismatic effect, it is sometimes necessary to prescribe a separate near glass appropriately decentered for near even in nonpresbyopes. Most patients, however, probably learn to move their heads sufficiently to use the area of the lenses very close to the optical centers for all purposes when decentering has not been prescribed. Prismatic effects may be avoided by a patient if he moves his head to maintain gaze through the _____ of his lenses.

49. (1) 5.00
(2) +

(Use a regular trial lens set for this frame.)

50. Neutralize a +1.00 D spherical lens from the trial case with the appropriate lens. The apparent motion of the image of this +1.00 D lens before neutralization is (1) _____. The neutralizing lens is (2) _____ D and is of (3) _____ sign.

---

221. 16

---

222. An uncorrected hyperope of 1.00 D working at 14 inches may develop symptoms of presbyopia at age _____.

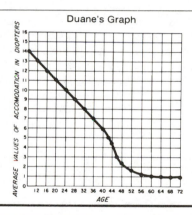

Duane's Graph

---

393. reduce the power of

---

394. To verify a proposed axis the handle of a cross cylinder is held and flipped while parallel to the proposed axis so that the axes of the cross cylinder are (1) _____ to the proposed
(at what angle)
axis. To check the power, the axes of the cross cylinder are placed and flipped over (2) _____ to the proposed cylinder.
(at what angle)

565. 170 degrees *(Record on data sheet; see Fig. 7.)*

---

566. With the axis determined, the power of the cylinder is tested by holding the cross cylinder with an axis (parallel to/45 degrees from) the axis of the cylinder in the trial frame.

---

737. (1) 1.5Δ   (3) 1.5Δ
     (2) down (4) up

---

738. Clinical experience indicates that only exceptionally do heterophorias require special correction other than correction of refractive errors. Indeed, exophoria may increase in amount if prisms are worn. Prisms are specifically not prescribed to correct _____ because of the tendency for this phoria to increase when so treated.

---

909. optical centers

---

910. Prismatic power for treatment of heterophoria may be induced by decentering the optical centers of the lenses. If base out prisms are desired for correction of an esophoria, they may be provided by decentering plus lenses in which direction?

50. (1) against
    (2) 1.00
    (3) −

(Use a regular trial lens set for this frame.)

51. Inspect the 0.00 lens from the auxiliary lenses. The apparent motion of the image is (1) _____ which indicates the power is (2) _____ .

---

222. 32

223. The age of onset of presbyopia is related not only to the amplitude of accommodation and the uncorrected refractive state of the eye but also to the habits of the individual. An illiterate laborer can be expected to develop symptoms of presbyopia much later than a Biblical scholar. Presbyopia is thus a relative term. The factors to be considered in diagnosing presbyopia are not age, but (1) _____ , (2) _____ , and (3) _____ .

---

394. (1) at 45 degrees
    (2) parallel

395. To refine the axis of a proposed minus cylinder using a cross cylinder it is usually best to move it in (1) _____ degree steps until the patient reports equal vision in both positions of the cross cylinder. Then test the power of the cylinder changing by (2) _____ D steps until equal vision with each of the two positions of the cross cylinder is again obtained.

566. parallel to

---

567. Cross cylinder tests for power of astigmatism depend upon the principle of contraction and expansion of the conoid of Sturm. Expanding the conoid results in an increase in the diameter of the circle of least confusion and hence increased blur of vision. Decreased blur of vision occurring when astigmatic power is being tested with cross cylinders indicates (1) _____ of the conoid of Sturm and (2) _____ in the diameter of the circle of least confusion.

---

738. exophoria

---

739. Esophoria at distance does not usually produce symptoms, but esophoria at near may. Patient A has 8Δ E and patient B has 8Δ E'. Which patient is more likely to have symptoms due to heterophoria?

---

910. out (laterally or temporally)

---

911. Decentering of a lens is not apparent without the use of a lensometer or other centering device, since the geometric center of the lens will coincide with the center of the patient's pupil in all cases. When the term decentration is used it is with reference to the _____ center of the lens and not the geometric.

51. (1) nil
     (2) zero

52. By convention, the meridians of an ophthalmic lens are numbered from 0 to 180 degrees, with 0 at the 3 o'clock position and counter-clockwise progression to 180 degrees when the lens is viewed from the front. On the diagram, the unnumbered heavy line indicates the _____ degrees meridian of the lens.

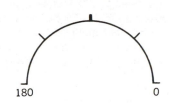

180   0

---

223. (1) uncorrected refractive error ⎫ in
     (2) amplitude of accommodation ⎬ any
     (3) vocation and avocation ⎭ order

224. Convergence is the simultaneous inturning of the eyes to maintain alignment of each visual axis with an object of regard closer to the eyes than 20 feet. A specific amount of convergence is required for a given eye to object distance. One method of measuring convergence is by the meter angle (ma). The amount of convergence required to maintain binocular fixation at a given distance may be expressed in _____.

---

395. (1) five
     (2) 0.25

396. The plus cylinder formula for a 0.50 D cross cylinder is $-0.50 + 1.00 \times$ any. For a 1.00 D cross cylinder it is $-1.00 + 2.00 \times$ any. Write the plus cylinder formula for a 0.25 D cross cylinder.

567. (1) contraction (or shortening)

(2) decrease

568. The lenses before OS patient A are -1.00 -1.50×170. The 0.25 D cross cylinder is held with minus axis parallel to 170 degrees (position 1) and then plus axis parallel to 170 degrees (position 2). The patient notes that numbers appear clearer with position 1 than with position 2, indicating that the minus cylinder should be (decreased/increased).

739. B

740. Since the amplitudes of vertical fusions are small, much smaller vertical heterophorias than horizontal produce symptoms. Vertical heterophorias of greater than 2Δ are rare, however, and prescription of prism base up or down is therefore equally rare. An RH of 6Δ is (1) (more/less) likely to produce symptoms than 6Δ E and will be found in patients (2) (more/less) often.

911. optical

912. In order for a lens to correct an optical defect in the eye, the back focal point of the lens must correspond to the far point of the eye. In spectacle lenses, which are optically "thick" lenses, the posterior focal length (or back vertex power) is of primary importance and is not necessarily the same as the anterior focal length. In the drawing, A is the (1) _____ of the eye and the (2) _____ of the lens.

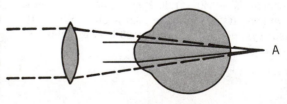

52. 90

---

53. Spherical lenses have the same power in all meridians. A lens in which the power varies from meridian to meridian is called a cylindrical lens, or cylinder for short. A lens with zero power at 180 degrees and +3.00 D power at 90 degrees is called a +3.00 D _____ lens.

---

224. meter angles (ma)

---

225. Convergence in meter angles is the reciprocal of the distance in meters from the eyes to the object of regard. An object viewed 1 m from the eyes requires _____ ma of convergence to maintain binocular fixation.

---

396. $-0.25 + 0.50 \times$ any

---

397. Write the minus cylinder formula for a 0.25 D cross cylinder.

568. increased

569. In the verification of astigmatic power with a cross cylinder the circle of least confusion must be _____ the retina.

740. (1) more
(2) less

741. Despite your conviction that prisms are not necessary for a given patient, if he has been wearing prisms in his most recent spectacles, it is inadvisable to eliminate them from a new correction. Your new prescription for a patient who has been wearing 2Δ base in OU will include _____.

912. (1) far point
(2) posterior focal point
(back focal point)

913. Since the posterior focal point of a lens is of primary importance in its ability to correct an optically imperfect eye, it follows that another lens of different power placed at a different position would be equally effective in correcting the error. Lenses which will correct the refractive error when placed at different locations before the eye are said to have equal effective powers. Lens A and B have the same _____.

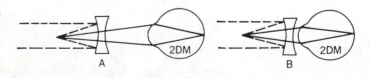

53. cylindrical

---

54. A cylindrical lens has a principal axis. Cylinders with a plane surface on one side are derivatives of cylindrical tubes. Consider a cylindrical tube with the axis of 45 degrees. Along this 45 degree axis there are no curves. All curves are perpendicular to 45 degrees, that is, at _____ degrees.

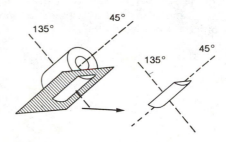

---

225. 1

---

226. Accommodation and convergence are directly, though flexibly, related. 1.00 D of accommodation and 1 ma of convergence are required for a pair of eyes with no refractive error to view an object at one meter binocularly. At 0.5 m viewing distance (1) _____ D of accommodation and (2) _____ ma of convergence are required for binocular clear vision.

---

397. $+0.25 - 0.50 \times$ any

---

398. The minus cylinder formula for a 0.25 D cross cylinder is $+0.25 - 0.50 \times$ any; for a 0.50 D cross cylinder it is $+0.50 - 1.00 \times$ any. Write the minus cylinder formula for a 0.75 D cross cylinder.

569. on

---

570. If −0.50 D cylinder is added to the combination of lenses before OS of patient A, _____ sphere must also be added to keep the circle of least confusion on the retina.

---

741. 2Δ base in (or prisms)

---

742. Psychogenic causes are frequently responsible for symptoms similar to asthenopia and those caused by heterophoria. Students and young homemakers are particularly prone to these psychogenic complaints which are usually periodic and of brief duration. Caution must be used to avoid prescribing insignificant corrections and prisms for patients in this category. If a student has symptoms related to use of his eyes in the presence of insignificant refractive error and heterophoria, the chances are they are _____ in origin.

---

913. effective power

---

914. If the position of a correcting lens is moved, its effective power changes. If a minus lens is moved closer to the eye as diagrammed, its effective minus power (increases/decreases) so that A and B coincide.

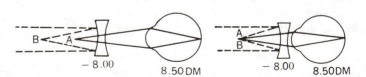

A = far point of eye
B = posterior focal point of lens

54. 135

---

55. The maximum curvature of cylinders is 90 degrees away from their axis. If the axis of the plus cylinder is 45 degrees, then the maximum curvature is at 135 degrees. If the minus cylinder axis is 30 degrees, the maximum curvature of this cylinder is at _____ degrees.

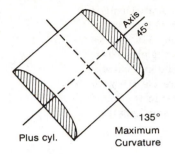

Axis 45°

135°
Maximum
Curvature

Plus cyl.

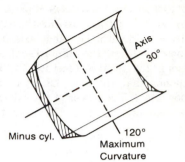

Axis 30°

120°
Maximum
Curvature

Minus cyl.

---

226. (1) 2.00
(2) 2

---

227. Convergence which is present as a result of accommodation is termed accommodative convergence. At any given distance a person with no refractive error exerts an equal amount of accommodation expressed in diopters and accommodative convergence expressed in _____.

---

398. $+0.75 - 1.50 \times$ any

---

399. To review the method of subjective refraction using astigmatic dials:
   Both ends of the conoid of Sturm are brought in front of the retina by fogging with (1) (minus/plus) (2) (spherical/cylindrical) lenses.

570. +0.25 D

---

571. The lenses before OS of patient A are changed to $-0.75 - 2.00 \times 170$ and the 0.25 D cross cylinder is held with the minus axis along 170 degrees (position 1) and then flipped so that the plus axis is along 170 degrees (position 2). The patient responds that the test characters are clearer with position 2. The power of the cylinder in the frame is therefore _____ than the astigmatism.

---

742. psychogenic

---

743. For comfort doing near tasks, a patient should have _____ percent of his accommodation in reserve.

---

914. increases

---

915. If a plus lens is moved away from the eye, its effective power _____ so that A and B coincide.

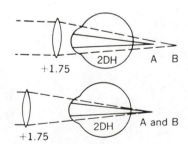

---

55. 120

---

56. Just as prisms do not displace lines perpendicular to their apices, so cylinders do not cause apparent motion of lines perpendicular to their axes. The power and sign of a cylinder are demonstrated by noting the apparent motion of a line _____ to its axis.

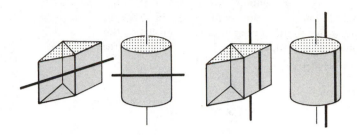

---

227. meter angles

---

228. Three meter angles of accommodative convergence accompany _____ D of accommodation.

---

399. (1) plus
(2) spherical

---

400. The second step in refraction using astigmatic dials is to move the conoid of Sturm posteriorly, bringing the posterior end of the conoid nearer the retina. This is done by decreasing the power of the (1) (plus/minus) spherical lenses to reduce the fog until the vision is about 20/70 if the astigmatism is large or about (2) _____ if the astigmatism is small.

571. greater (more)

---

572. Equal blur of test characters with each position of the cross cylinder when power is being tested indicates that the resulting conoid of Sturm is the same length in each position, and hence the circle of least confusion is _____ diameter in each position.

---

743. 50

---

744. Amplitude of accommodation _____ as age increases.

---

915. increases

---

916. The change in effective power as the position of a lens is altered is calculated from the power of the lens and the distance the lens is moved. Change in power = (change of distance in meters) × (power in diopters)^2 or $\Delta D = sD^2$.

A +10.00 D lens is moved 5 mm (0.005 m) closer to an eye. Its effective power decreases by _____ .

56. parallel

57. Since a cylinder has curvature along one meridian, it will converge or diverge light rays depending on whether it is convex or concave.

Light rays from a point source will be converged by a convex vertical cylinder to a (vertical/horizontal) line focus.

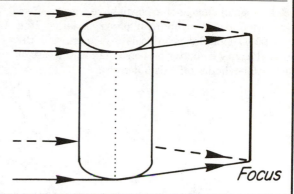

Focus

228. 3.00

229. The flexibility of the relationship between accommodative convergence and accommodation permits a variable accommodation while convergence is fixed, and vice versa. The amount of accommodation it is possible to exert above or below a fixed amount of convergence is termed relative accommodation. An individual utilizing 5.00 D of accommodation and 3 ma of convergence is exerting _____ D relative accommodation.

400. (1) plus
       (2) 20/40

401. After suitable fogging is achieved for the use of astigmatic dials the patient looks at an astigmatic dial and picks the (1) _____ line (or groups of lines). If a clock dial with lines every 30 degrees is used, the lower numbered hour indicating the blackest line is multiplied by (2) _____ to give the minus cylinder axis.

572. of equal (or the same)

---

573. A small change of axis will have a great effect in vision if the cylindrical power is large. If a −3.00 D cylinder is off axis 5 degrees, will the visual acuity be better or worse than in the case of a −0.50 cylinder off axis 5 degrees?

---

744. decreases

---

745. When reserve accommodation falls below 50 percent due to increasing age, the symptoms of _____ appear.

---

916. 0.50 D

---

917. A +10.00 lens moved 5 mm closer to an eye has lost 0.50 D in effective power, hence a stronger lens must be substituted to have the same effective power at the nearer position. A different lens placed at this location (5 mm closer than the original position of the +10.00 D lens) must have a power of _____ D to correct the eye.

57. vertical

58. The focal line produced by a cylinder is (perpendicular/ parallel) to the cylinder's axis.

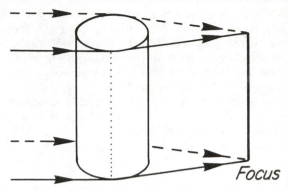

Focus

229. 2.00

230. Relative accommodation in excess of convergence is termed positive, while less than convergence is termed negative. The individual utilizing 5.00 D of accommodation and 3 ma of convergence is exerting 2.00 D of _____ relative accommodation.

401. (1) blackest
(2) 30

402. The next step in the correction of astigmatism using dials is to eliminate the conoid of Sturm. The patient looks at Lancaster Chart No. 2 (two perpendicular lines on a wheel which can be rotated). The wheel is turned so that one of the lines is _____ to the blacker line of the astigmatic dial and minus cylinders of increasing power are placed before the eye at the axis perpendicular to the blacker line.

573. Worse

574. Lenses before OS of patient A are changed to $-1.00 - 1.75 \times 170$. The 0.12 D change in the position of the circle of least confusion this entails is within the margins of error and may be ignored. The 0.25 D cross cylinder is held with minus axis parallel to 170 degrees (position 1) and then plus axis parallel to 170 degrees (position 2). Compare the two positions as illustrated. The power of the cylinder in the trial frame _____ the amount of astigmatism.

| $\frac{20}{30}$ | E D F C Z P | $\frac{30\text{ FT.}}{9.14\text{ M}}$ **6** |

1

| $\frac{20}{30}$ | E D F C Z P | $\frac{30\text{ FT.}}{9.14\text{ M}}$ **6** |

2

---

745. presbyopia

746. The need for special correction for presbyopia depends not only on the patient's age but also on his refractive state and habits of using his eyes. In addition to measuring a patient's amplitude of accommodation and assessing his habits of eye usage, it is necessary to determine his _____ before prescribing for presbyopia.

---

917. $+10.50$

918. The distance from the eye to the back surface of the lens is known as the vertex distance. If the vertex distance of a -12.00 D lens is increased 4 mm, its effective power (1) (increases/decreases) by (2) _____ D.

58. parallel

(Use a regular trial lens set for this frame.)

59. From the cylindrical lenses take a +2.00 D (cylindrical convex) lens. Small etched marks denote the axis. Align the axis with a vertical object. Note the movement of the image when the lens is moved perpendicular to these marks.

This (1) _____ movement reveals the effect on an image (2) (parallel/perpendicular) to the axis of the cylinder.

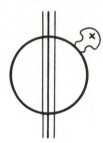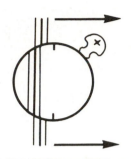

---

230. positive

---

231. Positive relative accommodation is measured by the strongest concave lenses through which an object at a fixed distance can be seen clearly binocularly (without diplopia). A patient with no refractive error who sees an object at 33 cm clearly and binocularly through concave lenses of increasing strength until the power of the lenses just exceeds −3.00 D has exerted _____ D of positive relative accommodation.

---

402. parallel (or perpendicular)

---

403. When the patient reports the 12-6 line the blackest, the axis of the correcting minus cylinder will be (6 × 30) 180 degrees. Correcting minus cylinders are always placed _____ to the blackest line on the astigmatic dial. This is the basis of the rule of 30.

574. equals

575. With the astigmatism neutralized, the conoid of Sturm has been changed to a _____ focus.

---

746. refractive state

747. If presbyopic correction is indicated, the correction should enable the patient to keep 50 percent of his _____ in reserve at his usual working distance.

---

918. (1) decreases
(2) 0.50 ($12 \times 12 \times 0.004 = 0.576$)

919. The formula $\Delta D = sD^2$ is used to calculate changes in (1) _____ of a lens when the (2) _____ is changed.

59. (1) against

(2) parallel

(Use a regular trial lens for this frame.)

60. Move this same +2.00 D cylinder (cylindrical convex) lens in the direction of the axis and observe the apparent motion of a horizontal line.

You have observed (1) _____ motion indicating that there (2) (is/is no) effect on an image perpendicular to the axis.

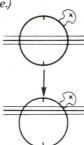

---

231. 3.00

---

232. Negative relative accommodation requires relaxation of accommodation and is determined by the strongest convex lenses through which an object at a fixed distance can be seen clearly binocularly. If these lenses measure +2.00 D a patient with no refractive error has _____ D of negative relative accommodation at that distance.

---

403. perpendicular

---

404. As minus cylinders are added in refraction using dials, (1) _____ D of plus sphere should be added with every (2) _____ D of minus cylinder to assure that the conoid of Sturm lies in front of the retina.

575. point

---

576. With $-1.00 - 1.75 \times 170$ before OS of patient A, the visual acuity is $20/15 - 2$. A -0.25 D sphere is added and the visual acuity remains the same but the patient observes a decrease in apparent size of the characters on the $20/15$ line of the Snellen chart. The patient has begun to _____.

---

747. accommodation

---

748. The initial symptoms of presbyopia are apt to appear at the end of the working day and when a patient attempts to read unusually small print or sew in poor light. Squinting, bright light, and lengthening of the reading distance will relieve these symptoms which are usually intermittent blurring, drowsiness, or asthenopia. Intermittent blurring of near vision at the end of the working day is a symptom of _____.

---

919. (1) effective power
(2) vertex distance

---

920. Write the formula for calculating change in effective power of a lens as vertex distance is changed.

60. (1) no
  (2) is no

61. A minus cylindrical lens can be generated from a tube. Consider a cylinder from a tube at axis 90 degrees.

There are no curves along axis 90 degrees, hence there is _____ net curvature along 90 degrees.

232. 2.00

233. Relative accommodation in excess of convergence is (1) _____ , and relative accommodation less than convergence is (2) _____ .

404. (1) 0.25
  (2) 0.50

405. As the final step in refraction with dials, the true or created myopia (which is now simple myopia instead of compound myopic astigmatism as it was before the conoid of Sturm was eliminated) is changed to emmetropia by reducing the amount of (1) _____ spheres until the next (2) _____ D change does not improve the acuity.

576. accommodate

---

577. The point focus in OS of patient A should be on the retina if the circle of least confusion has, as we assumed, been there. It is necessary to verify this by the addition of plus and minus spheres. A +0.25 D sphere is added to the correction and the visual acuity decreases to 20/20 − 3 from 20/15 − 2. This indicates that the point focus has been moved _____ to the retina.

---

748. presbyopia

---

749. The initial correction for presbyopia will be used only intermittently for near work, when the demands on accommodation are excessive, or when fatigue temporarily reduces the amplitude of accommodation. Presbyopia requiring an add up to +1.00 D is considered early presbyopia and corrections of this nature will generally be used only _____ for near work.

---

920. $\Delta D = sD^2$ [or (change in power) = (distance moved in meters) X (power in diopters)^2]

---

921. Vertex distance is extremely important in the case of high-powered lenses. The effect of moving a 10.00 D lens 5 mm is 0.50 D, whereas the same change in position of 2.00 D lens alters the effective power only 0.02 D. When strong plus or minus lenses are being prescribed, the _____ during refraction should be specified.

61. no (or 0)

---

62. A clue to the axis of the cylinder is the continuity of a vertical line as the lens is rotated.

The line rotates with the lens on the (−) minus axis. The minus axis can be accurately noted when an observed line is (continuous/rotated).

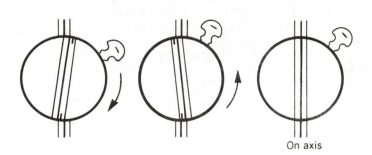

On axis

---

233. (1) positive relative accommodation
(2) negative relative accommodation

---

234. Negative relative accommodation is that amount of accommodation which can be relaxed while holding convergence fixed on a given distance and object. The negative relative accommodation is measured by the strongest _____ lenses through which a patient is able to maintain clear binocular vision at a given near distance.

---

405. (1) plus
(2) 0.25

---

406. The verification of the astigmatic correction by cross cylinders can only be done with the circle of least confusion on the retina. The fog is reduced to just best vision (before/after) the use of cross cylinders.

577. anterior

---

578. The final correction before OS of patient A has been found to be $-1.00 - 1.75 \times 170$. *(Record on data sheet; Fig. 7.)* This indicates an error in retinoscopy in determining (1) _____ and (2) _____ of the cylinder. *(Refer to Fig. 7.)*

---

749. intermittently

---

750. Near correction may be either in the form of single vision spectacles or bifocals. If a single vision near correction is prescribed, distance vision will be _____ while the patient is wearing it.

---

921. vertex distance

---

922. Since the back vertex power of a spectacle lens is of primary significance in refraction, distance spectacles being measured on the Lensometer are so placed that the temples are directed away from the examiner. In this way the _____ vertex power is determined.

62. continuous

63. The axis of a plus cylindrical lens can be determined by rotating the lens. A meridian just off the axis will be characterized by an apparent _____ motion with rotation of the lens.

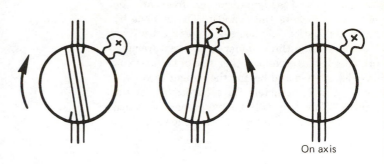

On axis

234. convex (plus)

235. Positive relative accommodation and negative relative accommodation should be about equal to permit comfort at a given working distance. A patient who has 3.00 D positive relative accommodation at a given distance and is comfortable at that distance would be expected to have about _____ D negative relative accommodation at the same distance.

406. before

407. The astigmatic correction can be checked with the cross cylinder. To check axis, the cross cylinder's axes are placed (1) _____ degrees to the proposed axis. The proposed minus cylindrical axis is rotated toward the (2) (plus/minus) cross cylinder axis with the cross cylinder in the position in which clearer vision is reported. The axis of the proposed cylinder is changed 5 degrees until vision with the cross cylinder in both positions is reported (3) _____.

578. (1) power ⎫ either
      (2) axis ⎭ order

---

579. The axis of astigmatism can frequently be verified by rocking the cylinder. This is done by asking the patient to observe a specific few test characters while the cylinder in the trial frame is rotated a few degrees to either side of the axis you have determined and having the patient report the clarity of the characters for each position of the cylinder. This test will be more sensitive when the power of the cylinder is (greater/lower).

---

750. blurred

---

751. Since corrections for early presbyopia will be used only occasionally, the advantages of a bifocal with an add less than +1.25 D will not be apparent to the patient, and a single vision lens should be prescribed. Since the far point through a weak add is relatively remote, he will not be certain through which portion of the bifocal, distance or near, he is looking. For early presbyopia either give a _____ near correction or wait until the presbyopia increases and a bifocal with an add of +1.25 or more is needed.

---

922. back

---

923. When measuring the power of the add of a fused bifocal, it is necessary, because of manufacturing techniques, to compare the front vertex power in the distance portion of the lens with the front vertex power in the segment portion. The spectacles will be in the lens power measuring device with the temples directed toward the examiner. The power of the fused bifocal segment is calculated with reference to the _____ power of the distance portion of the bifocal.

63. against

---

64. The phenomenon of clockwise or counterclockwise displacement does not occur with spherical lenses. Thus, when this phenomenon is present you know that you are looking through a _____ lens.

---

235. 3.00

---

236. A patient with no refractive error has 4.00 D negative relative accommodation at a given distance. This patient's positive relative accommodation would have to be about _____ at this same distance to permit comfortable work without glasses.

---

407. (1) 45
    (2) minus
    (3) equal (or equally blurred)

---

408. The power of the cylinder is checked by placing the cross cylinder's axes (1) _____ to the proposed axis. If the minus cross cylinder axis is parallel to the proposed axis in the position in which clearer vision is noted, (2) _____ cylinder is required; if the plus cross cylinder axis is parallel to the proposed axis, (3) _____ is required.

579. greater

---

580. A technique for verification of cylinder axis which requires the patient to note the clarity of test characters as a cylinder is moved to various axes in the trial frame known as _____.

---

751. single vision

---

752. Myopes with a far point at a convenient working distance and without undue astigmatism will generally not require separate correction for early presbyopia since removal of the distance correction will achieve the desired result. When, as accommodation decreases, this becomes inconvenient because of the frequency with which it must be done, bifocals are indicated. In early presbyopia many myopes will be comfortable if they _____ whenever necessary for near work.

---

923. front vertex

---

924. During refraction the strongest spherical lens being used is placed in the _____ of the trial frame.

64. cylindrical

(Use a regular trial lens set for this frame.)

65. Every cylinder has a minus and a plus cylinder axis. Later you will learn how to transpose a minus cylinder lens formula onto a plus cylinder form. Using a −2.00 D cylindrical lens from the trial case, observe the rotational displacement of a line perpendicular to the minus axis. This rotational displacement is (1) (with/against), and demonstrates the (2) (plus/minus) axis.

---

236. 4.00 D

---

237. At the near point of accommodation (where any minus lens will cause a blur, since the patient is using maximal accommodation) an individual has _____ D positive relative accommodation.

---

408. (1) parallel (or perpendicular)
    (2) minus
    (3) plus cylinder (or less minus cylinder)

---

409. The near astigmatic correction is slightly different from the distance correction, if carefully measured. The reasons for this are:

(a) The ciliary muscle probably is not exactly uniform.
(b) The lens density and capsule densities are not uniform.
(c) The eye torts (vertical axis turns) slightly as patient converges on a near object.

While the above are true they are disregarded and the distance astigmatic correction is usually prescribed for near as well as for distance.

Is the near astigmatic error customarily measured? (1) _____.

If the near astigmatism measures a different amount and axis than the distance astigmatism you will use the (2) (near/distant) astigmatism in the final prescription.

580. rocking the cylinder

581. Automated refractors have been developed with which a patient can be subjectively or objectively refracted. Automated refractors require relatively clear ocular media for accuracy. Patients with moderately advanced cataracts (are/are not) good candidates for automated refractors.

752. remove their distance glasses

753. Patients become more dependent upon their near correction as the amplitude of accommodation continues to decrease. When the necessary add is +1.25 D or more, virtually all tasks at the average near working distance demand use of the near correction, and it is logical to recommend bifocals to a patient. Bifocals are usually recommended for presbyopes when the required add is _____ or more.

924. back cell

925. Trial lenses are so designed that the total power of the combination of any spherical lens and cylindrical lens is specified as the back vertex power of the lens closest to the eye, provided that the sphere is placed closer to the eye and the cylinder and sphere are oriented the same way. This design enables a single spectacle lens to be prescribed with a back vertex power equivalent to the power of the combination in the trial frame. The power of a cylinder in the trial set is expressed in respect to the _____ of any sphere in the back cell of the trial frame.

65. (1) against
    (2) plus

---

66. Combinations of spheres and cylinders may be generated as from a doughnut. The curve with the larger radius will be the circumference of the doughnut. Perpendicular to this and parallel to the diameter of the doughnut will be the curve with the shorter radius. This resultant lens has plus power in both meridians. The higher power is located along the shorter radius, hence at (1) _____ degrees and the axis of this higher power is 90 degrees away, located at (2) _____ degreees.

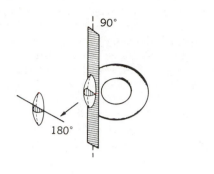

---

237. zero

---

238. In order to see clearly at 20 cm an emmetropic eye (an eye with no refractive error) must accommodate _____ D.

---

409. (1) No (except for research purposes or your interest)
    (2) distant

---

410. It is common to find large amounts of astigmatism. A good rule to follow is to give the full amount of cylinder found in all children. In adults one should be cautious. If the astigmatism is with the rule, be especially hesitant to give the full cylinder. Frequently give one quarter or one half and a year later increase the cylinder. In astigmatism against the rule, the cylinder may be given a little more liberally, always remembering that some adults have a difficult time adjusting to any new condition and a new cylinder creates a new world.

With the rule astigmatism should be slightly (under/over) corrected as compared to against the rule astigmatism.

581. are not

---

582. Subjective automated refractors require focus adjustments by the patient whose performance must be monitored by a technician. The instruments have adjustable vertex distance (distance between eye and lens) and a method of relaxing accommodation. In addition some of them are able to test binocular functions. The more functions measured, the more adjustments required of the patient. Intellectually impaired patients (are/are not) good candidates for automated subjective refractors.

---

753. +1.25 D

---

754. Discomfort in bright light, both indoors and out, is not an infrequent complaint. Spectacle manufacturers provide glass lenses in a variety of tints, including some which vary depending upon the amount of incident ultraviolet. Plastic lenses are easily surface tinted by an optician. Fashion trends often dictate a patient's decision to have tinted glasses. All tints reduce the total amount of light entering the eye. A patient's real or imagined discomfort to light may be reduced by _____ his glasses.

---

925. back vertex power

---

926. In addition to placing the sphere in the back cell of the trial frame, for trial lens combinations to be truly additive, it is necessary that they be oriented surface to surface as specified. This means that for each lens used the figure on the handle indicating power should be facing the examiner. If the lenses in the trial frame are reversed front to back, they are no longer truly _____ .

66. (1) 180
   (2) 90

---

67. A lens surface having two radii of curvature is called a toric surface.

A lens with + 3.00 D at 90 degrees and + 6.00 D at 180 degrees is a spherocylindrical or _____ lens.

---

238. 5.00

---

239. Accommodative spasm is the continued expenditure of accommodation in excess of the normal requirement, with the result that the far point and near point of the eyes are brought closer to the patient. An emmetrope who has spasm of accommodation becomes _____ .

---

410. under

---

411. A progressive bulging of the cornea, called **keratoconus**, produces progressive astigmatism. The cornea in keratoconus becomes thin and may even rupture, so its physical condition must be followed with care. Contact lenses are usually used, since some of the astigmatism is frequently irregular. If the condition continues to worsen a corneal graft is indicated. A progressive thinning of the cornea with increasing astigmatism is called _____ .

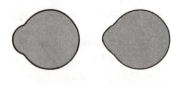

Normal   Keratoconus

582. are not

---

583. The results of an objective automated refractor should be the same as that arrived at by retinoscopy. Just as retinoscopy findings need refinement, whenever possible, so must the automated refractor data be verified and refined. The displayed data of an automated refractor should be used similarly to _____.

---

754. tinting

---

755. Patients with cataracts have an impediment to the passage of light into the eye. Tinted glasses reduce the transmission of light. A patient with cataracts (should/should not) use tinted glasses at night.

---

926. additive

---

927. Trial lens design provides that spherocylindrical combinations may be expressed as the back vertex power of a single equivalent lens provided the trial lenses are placed in the trial frame with the sphere in the (1) _____ and the surfaces of the trial lenses are oriented in the (2) _____ direction.

67. toric

(Use a regular trial lens set for this frame.)

68. Place a +2.00 D sphere and a +2.00 D cylinder together with the axis of the cylinder at 90 degrees.

The apparent movement of the image when the lenses are moved up and down or sideways is _____.

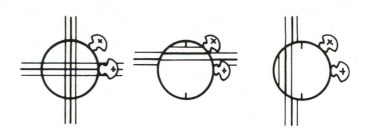

---

239. myopic

---

240. The continued excess of accommodation in spasm of accommodation is the result of spasm of the ciliary muscles. Spasm of accommodation can therefore be eliminated by _____ drugs.

---

411. keratoconus

---

412. Any changing astigmatism should be viewed with suspicion. If a tumor presses on the back of the eye, the fovea may be distorted and astigmatism result. A tumor indenting the back of the eye would probably make the eye (myopic/hyperopic) as well as astigmatic.

583. retinoscopy findings

---

584. The amplitudes of accommodation of the two eyes are usually _____.

---

755. should not

---

756. Medical reasons for prescribing tinted glasses are rare. Generally, therefore, a patient may make his own decisions about tints. Tinted glasses to be used at night, however, are contraindicated for patients with _____.

---

927. (1) back cell
    (2) same

928.

PART XII

CONTACT LENSES

(Advance to next frame.)

68. against

(Use a regular trial lens set for this frame.)

69. Rotate this same combination ($+2.00 \smile +2.00 \times 90$ degrees) back and forth, noting the apparent motion of a vertical line.

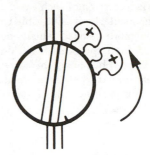

The motion of the image is (1) _____ the rotation of the lenses. This motion indicates the axis of the (2) _____ cylinder.

---

240. cycloplegic

---

241. Accommodative spasm results in the development of myopia in an emmetrope, or the worsening of existing myopia. Either condition is called pseudomyopia. Pseudomyopia is caused by _____ .

---

412. hyperopic

---

413. The uniformity of corneal curves may be conveniently tested with a **Placido disc** or a self-illuminated Placido disc called a **keratoscope**. The principle is that a uniform spherical surface will reflect concentric rings uniformly. If the sphere is not uniform, as in keratoconus, the concentric circles will be distorted. Which image, A or B, indicates keratoconus?

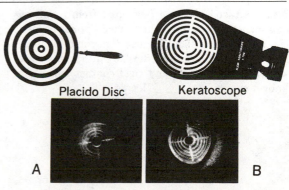

Placido Disc   Keratoscope

A   B

584. equal

---

585. A source of discomfort in wearing spectacles is unequal accommodative demand on the two eyes. With the refractive error of each eye having been determined monocularly, it is possible that accommodation was more relaxed when one eye was being refracted than the other. Checking for this possibility is termed balancing the correction. If it has been determined that accommodation was equally relaxed as each eye was refracted, the correction is said to be _____ .

---

756. cataracts

757.

PART X

PRESBYOPIA AND BIFOCALS

(*Advance to next frame.*)

---

928. (*Advance to next frame.*)

---

929. Contact lenses are fabricated from a variety of synthetic materials which have optical properties approaching those of glass. They may be flexible (soft) or rigid (hard). Flexible contact lenses are known as soft lenses and rigid contact lenses are known as _____ lenses.

69. (1) opposite (or against)
(2) plus

---

70. All cylinders have a minus cylinder axis and a plus cylinder axis, and these two axes are always 90 degrees apart.

Regardless of the sign of the lens, *against* rotational displacement indicates the plus cylinder axis, and *with* rotational displacement indicates the minus cylinder axis.

If a lens is rotated clockwise and a clockwise (with) rotational displacement is discerned, this unknown lens is a cylindrical lens and the rotational displacement is occurring along the _____ cylinder axis.

---

241. spasm of accommodation (or spasm of the ciliary muscle)

---

242. Spasm of accommodation is generally functional and occurs primarily in children and young adults. If the condition is not severe and the accommodative amplitude large, the only symptom may be pseudomyopia. An otherwise asymptomatic child found to have 2.00 D of myopia when examined without cycloplegia and no myopia with cycloplegia is probably suffering from _____.

---

413. B

---

414. Just as astigmatism may be produced by indentation of the globe, so may changes in the retina, such as edema of the retina or elevation of one side of the macula by tumors, produce astigmatism.

If the retina is elevated eccentrically (displaced anteriorly), the eye will have increasing (1) _____ and (2) _____.

585. balanced

---

586. To balance the correction, a plus sphere of equal power (+0.62 D is convenient) is added to the final correction before each eye and the patient is permitted to view the Snellen chart binocularly for a few seconds. Each eye is briefly occluded and the patient is instructed to read the lowest line of Snellen letters he can easily see with the unoccluded eye. If the correction is balanced the vision of each eye should be _____.

---

757. (*Advance to next frame.*)

---

758. A decrease in the amplitude of accommodation in the emmetrope causes presbyopic symptoms to appear, usually between ages 40 and 45. These symptoms are blurring of small print at near, and attempting to hold material far enough away from the eyes to permit clearer vision.

Blurred near vision in a 45-year-old emmetrope is usually due to _____.

---

929. hard

---

930. Contact lenses rest on the surface of the cornea, separated from it by a film of tears. Since the tears have an index of refraction close to that of the cornea, the front surface of the cornea is eliminated as a refracting surface, and the front surface of the contact lens becomes, in effect, the anterior refracting surface of the eye. When a contact lens is worn, the anterior surface of the _____ is eliminated as a refracting surface.

70. minus

(Use a regular trial lens set for this frame.)

71. Rotate the same combination of lenses ($+2.00 \subset +2.00 \times 90$ degrees) in the manner diagrammed, and note the rotational image displacement of a horizontal line. This apparent (1) _____ rotation of the image indicates a (2) _____ cylinder axis.

---

242. pseudomyopia (or spasm of accommodation)

---

243. If the spasm of accommodation is severe or if the amplitude of accommodation is small in the presence of spasm of accommodation, near work may be difficult as well as distance vision blurred. Discomfort with near work or blurring of vision at near associated with myopia in a child should lead one to suspect _____.

---

414. (1) hyperopia   either
      (2) astigmatism   order

---

415. Unusual pressure from localized portions of the lids can produce astigmatism. The lids should be suspected as a cause for new astigmatism and they should be checked for chalazia (localized granulation) or tumors. Tumors of the lids usually squeeze the cornea vertically, causing astigmatism with the rule. This astigmatism will disappear when the tumors have been removed.

Lid tumors may cause (1) _____, and you would expect it to be (2) _____ the rule.

586. equal (or equally blurred)

---

587. In the case of patient A, a +0.62 D added to each eye results in a visual acuity in each eye of 20/40. The correction is _____ .

---

758. presbyopia

---

759. A decrease in the amplitude of accommodation may occur in conditions other than presbyopia such as (1) parasympathetic paralysis due to systemic drugs; (2) local ocular medication; (3) trauma to the eye; and (4) Adie's syndrome. What type of systemic medications would be expected to affect the amplitude of accommodation?

---

930. cornea

---

931. The anterior surface of a contact lens is, in effect, the anterior _____ surface of the eye.

71. (1) with
    (2) minus

---

72. The term **form** applied to an ophthalmic lens refers to its physical appearance in cross section. The term **shape** applied to an ophthalmic lens refers to its physical appearance as viewed from a point perpendicular to its surfaces, that is, from the front or back. The cross section on the right illustrates the _____ of a lens.

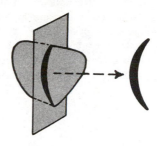

---

243. spasm of accommodation (or pseudomyopia)

---

244. Spasm of accommodation is a result of spasm of the _____ muscles.

---

415. (1) astigmatism
    (2) with

---

416. Since astigmatism is the result of different meridians having different refractive errors, if vision through all except one meridian is eliminated, a sphere can be used to measure the error in the isolated meridian.

The stenopaic slit is a movable slit which can be used to eliminate the astigmatic error and treat any meridian as only a spherical error. The refractive error of this eye would be: _____.

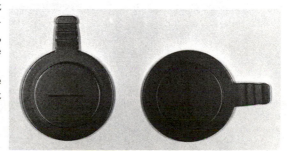

+2.00 = Refractive error
Position "A"

−5.00 = Refractive error
Position "B"

587. balanced

---

588. To balance a correction +0.62 D has been added to the distance correction before each eye. Visual acuity with the correction and without this add was 20/15 in each eye. Visual acuity with correction and +0.62 D added is 20/20 OD and 20/40 OS. This indicates that during the refraction _____ was more relaxed in OS than OD.

---

759. Parasympatholytic (or anticholinergic)

---

760. Adie's syndrome occurs most frequently in females and consists of a tonic pupil, decreased amplitude of accommodation, and reduced ankle or knee jerks.

A 30-year-old woman, who complains of blurred near vision OD, has a pupil which constricts slowly but fully to light and dilates slowly but completely in the dark, and who has absent ankle jerks, probably has _____.

---

931. refracting

---

932. The space between contact lens and cornea is filled by the _____.

72. form

---

73. The surface of a lens which is convex toward air is termed a plus curve and has plus power. That surface which is concave toward air is termed a minus curve and has minus power. In the drawing, the back surface of the lens (toward the eye) is (1) _____, and hence a (2) _____ curve.

---

244. ciliary

---

245. Spasm of accommodation may be associated with spasm of convergence and constriction of the pupils. This group of findings is known as spasm of the near reflex and is also generally functional. Spasm of the near reflex includes spasm of accommodation, (1) _____ and (2) _____ and is usually due to (3) _____ causes.

---

416. + 2.00 − 7.00 × 180
   (or − 5.00 + 7.00 × 90)

---

417. A clue to keratoconus or lenticonus is a dark circle when the red pupillary reflex is viewed from about 10 inches. This dark circle is simply the area of a change of curvature when the rays are projected away from your eye leaving a dark circle behind.

A dark circle in the pupillar reflex may indicate (1) _____ or (2) _____.

 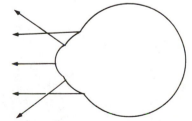

588. accommodation

589. If, with the balancing lenses added, a difference of visual acuity between the eyes of more than one Snellen line is present, additional plus is added to the eye with the better vision 0.25 D at a time until the blur equals that in the other eye. Vision with correction is 20/15 in each eye of a patient. Add of +0.62 D reduces the distance vision to 20/40 OD and 20/20 OS. Additional plus will be added to (1) _____ until the vision is reduced to (2) _____ .

760. Adie's syndrome

761. Patients with Adie's syndrome have reduced parasympathetic innervations of the involved eye and have an increased sensitivity to parasympathomimetics. One-sixteenth percent (0.0625%) pilocarpine has no effect on a normal eye but will cause miosis in the affected eye in Adie's syndrome.

To test for Adie's syndrome (1) _____ is instilled in both eye and miosis is expected in the (2) _____ eye.

932. tear film

933. Most astigmatism of the eye is due to toricity of the anterior surface of the _____ .

73. (1) concave
(2) minus

---

74. Lenses may be biconcave in form and have two
_____ curves toward the air.

---

245. (1) spasm of convergence ⎫ either
(2) constriction of the pupils ⎬ order
(3) functional ⎭

246.

PART III

CYCLOPLEGICS

(Advance to next frame.)

---

417. (1) keratoconus
(2) lenticonus

---

418. In contrast to keratoconus, the astigmatism
caused by lenticonus (a conical crystalline lens)
(can/cannot) be corrected with a contact lens.

589. (1) OS
(2) 20/40

590. A difference in vision between the eyes when balancing lenses have been added to the correction indicates that the eye with the (better/worse) vision was accommodating more during the refraction.

761. (1) pilocarpine 0.0625 percent
(2) affected

762. The cause of Adie's syndrome is unknown. Patients with this condition have been followed for over 20 years without developing any related or common disease. The loss of accommodation is frequently permanent. Adie's syndrome is associated with _____ systemic disease.

933. cornea

934. If the toric anterior surface of the cornea is covered by a spherical surfaced hard contact lens, the tear film neutralizes the _____ caused by the toricity of the corneal surface.

74. minus

---

75. Just as two minus curves give a biconcave lens form, so two plus curves, as illustrated, give a _____ lens form.

---

246. *(Advance to next frame.)*

---

247. The ciliary body is sometimes referred to as the circular muscle; hence the terms cyclitis for inflammation and cycloplegia for paralysis of the ciliary body. A drug paralyzing the ciliary muscle is a _____ drug.

---

418. cannot

419.

PART V

INTERPUPILLARY DISTANCE AND TRIAL FRAME

(Advance to next frame.)

590. better

---

591. In general, if a difference in relaxation of accommodation between the eyes during refraction has been demonstrated by balancing, the correction prescribed for one of the eyes is changed. The change is an amount equal to the difference in additional plus needed to produce equal blur. In a given patient $+1.12$ D added to the distance correction before one eye and $+0.62$ D before the other produces equal blur at distance. The prescribed correction before one eye will differ from that found before balancing by _____ D.

---

762. no

---

763. The loss of accommodation in Adie's syndrome may be annoying to the young patient. A weak solution of pilocarpine or other parasympathomimetic drug may cause miosis great enough to produce a pinhole effect and thus decrease the symptoms.

The symptoms of Adie's syndrome may be alleviated with a _____.

---

934. astigmatism

---

935. Spherical hard contact lenses eliminate _____ caused by toricity of the anterior surface of the cornea.

75. biconvex.

---

76. If one surface of a lens is flat and the other curved, the form is termed either plano (1) _____ or plano (2) _____ .

---

247. cycloplegic

---

248. Since contraction of the ciliary muscle results in accommodation, cycloplegic drugs produce _____ of accommodation.

---

419. (*Advance to next frame.*)

---

420. The interpupillary distance is usually termed the pupillary distance for P.D. More specifically, the P.D. is the distance between visual axes.

The P.D. is an abbreviation for the (1) _____ and is the distance between the (2) _____ .

591. 0.50

592.

	Correction before balancing	Balancing lens
OD	+1.00	+0.62
OS	−1.00	+1.12

Accommodation was more relaxed in which eye during refraction before balancing?

---

763. parasympathomimetic drug (or weak solution of pilocarpine)

---

764. Decreased amplitude of accommodation may be a complaint of patients receiving atropine or other parasympatholytic drugs.

A patient with a duodenal ulcer who is being treated medically might complain of blurred near vision. The cause of the presbyopic symptoms would probably be _____.

---

935. astigmatism

---

936. Soft contact lenses conform to a great extent with the shape of the anterior corneal surface. The anterior surface of a soft lens placed on a toric cornea will be a (toric/spherical) surface.

76. (1) convex ⎫ either
(2) concave ⎭ order

77. The form of lens A is (1) _____.
The form of lens B is (2) _____.

A   B

---

248. paralysis (or relaxation)

249. Cycloplegic drugs for refraction are instilled into the conjunctival sac in drop or ointment form. Cycloplegic drugs to be used for refraction are prescribed as (1) _____ or (2) _____.

---

420. (1) pupillary distance
(or interpupillary distance)
(2) visual axes

421. Any deviation of the optical center of a lens from the visual axis will result in prismatic effect. The direction of the prismatic effect will depend on the sign of the lens and the relation of the optical center of the lens to the _____.

592. OD

593.

	Correction before balancing	Total power to see 20 / 40	Full plus for 20 / 20	Prescribed, based on reducing plus OD
OD	+1.00	+1.62	+1.00	+0.50
OS	+1.00	+2.12	+1.50	+1.00

accommodated _____ during the refraction.

From the table, OS was accommodating more before balancing than OD and hence needs more plus to be fogged. In hyperopia the final prescription is the result of reducing plus in the eye which

---

764. systemic parasympatholytic drugs (such as atropine or belladonna)

---

765. The symptoms of decreased amplitude of accommodation due to systemic atropine usually occur in those patients whose amplitude of accommodation is poor and who would soon need a presbyopic correction.

A 20-year-old male receiving systemic atropine to reduce gastric acidity (would/would not) be expected to have blurred near vision due to the atropine.

---

936. toric

---

937. Soft lenses usually (do/do not) eliminate astigmatism caused by a toric anterior corneal surface.

77. (1) planoconvex
(2) planoconcave

---

78. Most ophthalmic lenses are ground in a **meniscus** form, as shown here. The front surface of a meniscus lens is (1) _____ and has (2) _____ power.

---

249. (1) drops ⎫ either
(2) ointment ⎭ order

---

250. The most effective cycloplegic drugs in common use are parasympatholytic. Of these, atropine results in the most profound cycloplegia. The parasympatholytic drug producing the greatest cycloplegia is _____ .

---

421. visual axis

---

422. The P.D. must be known in order to align the centers of the trial lenses with the visual axes. If the optical centers of the lenses coincide with the visual axes, the distance between the optical centers of the lenses must equal the _____ .

593. less

---

594. As a general rule, when balancing lenses are unequal the plus of the final prescription for hyperopia is reduced in the eye which had accommodation more relaxed during refraction. For example, a patient has a visual acuity of 20/15 in each eye with +1.00 D spheres OU. On balancing, an additional +0.62 OD gave 20/40 and an additional +1.12 OS gave 20/40. The final prescription will be OD _____ D and OS + 1.00 D.

---

765. would not

---

766. Loss of accommodation in the child or young adult is most frequently associated with the accidental instillation of a cycloplegic in the eye. Frequently just rubbing the eyelids after having touched a cycloplegic is sufficient to produce mydriasis and cycloplegia.

A 24-year-old nurse presents with uniocular mydriasis and loss of accommodation. The probable cause is _____.

---

937. do not

---

938. When soft contact lenses are worn, any significant _____ must be corrected by spectacles.

78. (1) convex
(2) plus

79. The back surface of a meniscus lens is (1) _____ and has (2) _____ power.

250. atropine

251. Scopolamine, homatropine, cyclopentolate, and tropicamide, like atropine, produce cycloplegia by the pharmacologic effect on the ciliary muscle known as _____.

422. P.D.

423. The visual axes are virtually parallel when a distant object is fixated. When a near object is viewed the eyes must converge (turn in) to allow both foveas to fixate the object.

The near P.D. is (greater/less) than the distance P.D.

594. +0.50

---

595. A patient has a visual acuity of 20/20 in each eye with +2.00 D spheres OU. On balancing an additional +0.62 gives 20/40 OD and +1.87 gives 20/40 OS. The correction prescribed will be OD (1) _____ and OS (2) _____.

---

766. accidental instillation of a cycloplegic in the eye (or rubbing the eyes after handling cycloplegic drugs)

---

767. The measurements of accommodation should be done binocularly through the balanced distance correction. Since the distant refraction brings both eyes to emmetropia, accommodative demands at near will be _____ for the two eyes.

---

938. astigmatism

---

939. Contact lenses may be used to correct any refractive error. High amounts of corneal astigmatism (> 3.00 D), however, make the fitting of spherical hard lenses difficult, and soft lenses generally (1) (do/do not) correct astigmatism. Corneal contact lenses are generally contraindicated in the presence of large amounts of corneal (2) _____.

79. (1) concave
(2) minus

80. If the powers of both surfaces of a lens are known, the total power of the lens may be estimated by algebraically adding the surface powers. The meniscus lens drawn has an approximate total power of _____ D.

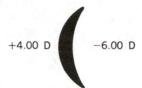

+4.00 D   −6.00 D

251. parasympatholytic

252. If a cycloplegic eliminates all accommodation, a patient will be able to read clearly print held _____ cm from the eye with a +3.00 D add over his distance correction.

423. less

424. You will remember that a meter angle is a unit of measure of convergence. Meter angles are calculated by dividing the distance (in centimeters) between the object of regard and the eyes into 100 (the reciprocal of the distance in meters).

An object at 50 cm requires 2 ma convergence for binocular fixation.

How many meter angles convergence are needed to fixate an object at 33.33 cm.?

595. (1) +0.75 D
(2) +2.00 D

---

596. If the patient is myopic the following would be an example of balancing and prescribing:

	Refraction	Total Balance for 20 / 40	20 / 20	Finax Rx
OD	−5.00	−4.37	−5.00	−5.00
OS	−5.00	−3.87	−4.50	−4.50

The table indicates that only the minus should be prescribed that is necessary to bring each eye to the best vision without stimulating _____ .

---

767. the same (or equal)

---

768. For comfort at a near working distance the amplitude of accommodation should be twice the demand. If the near work of the patient is to be done at 33.33 cm, the amplitude of accommodation should be at least _____ D.

---

939. (1) do not
(2) astigmatism

---

940. Irregular anterior corneal astigmatism may be corrected by a (soft/hard) contact lens.

160

80. -2.00

---

81. In spherical meniscus lenses the lower powered curve (either plus or minus) is called the base curve. The base curve of this lens is _____ D.

+8.00 D   −4.00 D

---

252. 33.33

---

253. Residual accommodation is the amount of accommodation remaining after a cycloplegic has been used. If a patient who has received a cycloplegic can read print clearly placed anywhere between 25 and 33.33 cm from his eye with a $+3.00$ D add over his distance correction, he has 1.00 D of _____ accommodation.

---

424. 3

---

425. Meter angles of convergence indicate the distance between the object of regard and the eyes. The degrees of convergence necessary for binocular fixation are dependent on this distance and the P.D. A large P.D. requires greater convergence than a small P.D. When an object 25 cm away from the eyes is fixated, (1) _____ ma of convergence are required. Convergence demands are greater for a (2) (small/large) P.D.

596. accommodation

---

597. As a general rule in myopia, when a change in correction is necessary to balance, the minus is reduced before the eye in which accommodation was more active during refraction. A patient has a visual acuity of 20/20 in each eye with −4.00 D sphere OU. On balancing an additional +0.62 gives 20/40 OD and an additional +1.37 gives 20/40 OS. The final correction is OD (1) _____ and OS (2) _____.

---

768. 6.00

---

769. If the near work of the patient is done at 50 cm, the amplitude of accommodation should be _____ D if the patient is to be comfortable.

---

940. hard

---

941. Despite the inability of soft lenses to correct anterior corneal astigmatism, they have proven superior to hard lenses for some patients because they are better tolerated by the cornea. Safer and more comfortable wearing for some patients is an advantage of (soft/hard) lenses.

81. -4.00

82. In this spherical lens -6.00 D is the _____ curve.

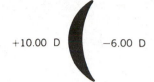

+10.00 D   −6.00 D

253. residual

254. Residual accommodation can be determined by placing a $+3.00$ D add over the distance correction and moving print first away from the eye and then toward the eye until it blurs in each case. If under these circumstances print is clear between 50 cm and 20 cm from the eye, the patient has _____ D residual accommodation.

425. (1) 4
      (2) large

426. Males usually have a wider P.D. than females, Blacks wider than Caucasians, and Orientals narrower than Caucasians.
   A Caucasian female would be expected to have a (wider/narrower) P.D. than a Black male.

597. (1) − 4.00

(2) − 3.25

---

598. The simple rule in balancing is to reduce plus in hyperopia and reduce minus in myopia. In hyperopia and myopia you do not prescribe a lens (greater/lesser) in power than that found in the prebalanced refraction.

---

769. 4.00

---

770. If the visual demands of the patient are carefully ascertained, the amplitude of accommodation necessary for the task is easily calculated. If the patient's near work is done primarily at 66.66 cm, his amplitude of accommodation should be _____ for him to be comfortable without a reading correction.

---

941. soft

---

942. Not all astigmatism is anterior corneal. Astigmatism produced by the anterior surface of the crystalline lens (is/is not) eliminated by spherical hard contact lenses.

82. base

---

83. Corrections for astigmatism require that a cylinder be ground on one or both sides of a lens. In ophthalmic lenses, the cylinder is ground on one side, creating a toric surface. The other surface of the lens remains (spherical/spherocylindrical).

---

254. 3.00

---

255. Residual accommodation is measured monocularly. Binocular measurement of residual accommodation (is/is not) satisfactory.

---

426. narrower

---

427. P.D. is measured in millimeters. Caucasian males' P.D.s vary from 58 to 72 mm and Caucasian females' P.D.s vary from 57 to 65 mm.

Many Black males have P.D.s (1) (wider/narrower) than 72 mm.

Many Oriental females might have P.D.s (2) (wider/narrower) than 57.

598. greater

599. Complete refraction includes a determination of muscle balance at distance and near with the new correction in the trial frame. In patient A the muscle balance will be tested at distance with the lenses (1) _____ before OD and (2) _____ before OS. *(Refer to data sheet; see Fig. 7.)*

770. 3.00 D

771. To determine whether or not the amplitude of accommodation is at least twice the demand, type or objects consistent with the visual demands are placed at the working distance as determined by the history. For comfort the patient should be able to accommodate at least two times the working distance. If the print is placed at 50 cm and the patient can still read this print through -2.00 D lenses OU placed over his distance correction, he has (1) _____ D of accommodation and (2) (needs/does not need) a reading correction.

942. is not

943. Astigmatism measureable when a spherical hard contact lens is being worn is termed "residual astigmatism." Residual astigmatism does not result from toricity of _____.

83. spherical

---

84. A meniscus lens which corrects astigmatism has one surface which is spherical, and one surface which is a combination of sphere and cylinder called a _____ surface.

---

255. is not

---

256. Residual accommodation may be measured by holding print at any reading distance and there determining the least and most amount of plus power over the distance correction with which the print can be clearly seen. An eye under cycloplegia cannot read print until an add of +2.25 D is placed before the eye. Print remains clear at that distance when a + 3.50 D add is placed before the eye. Any further plus lens causes the print to blur. The eye has _____ D residual accommodation.

---

427. (1) wider
(2) narrower

---

428. To measure the near P.D. hold a flashlight close to your left eye (closing your right) 14 inches in front of the patient. Have the patient look at the flashlight. Hold a millimeter (mm) rule in front of the patient (as close to the eyes as possible) so you can just see the center of the pupil above the rule. Align zero on the ruler with the corneal reflex (of the flashlight) of the patient's OD and read the near P.D. on the millimeter rule by noting the position of the corneal reflex OS.

This reading is a measurement of the _____ P.D.

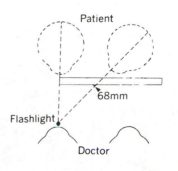

599. (1) $-1.00 - 1.00 \times 25$

     (2) $-1.00 - 1.75 \times 170$

600.

PART VIII

HETEROPHORIAS

(*Advance to next frame.*)

---

771. (1) 4.00

     (2) does not need

---

772. At 33.33 cm, the patient's working distance, he can read print through -1.00 D spheres added to his distance correction, but -1.25 D spheres blur him. He has 4 D of accommodation (3 D to see at 33.33 cm and 1 D to overcome -1.00 D lenses).

A patient who can read print at 25 cm through -1.00 D spheres added to his distance correction has _____ D accommodation.

---

943. the anterior corneal surface

---

944. On occasion an eye which can be corrected by a spherical spectacle lens is found to have residual astigmatism when a hard contact lens is worn. In this situation the cornea is found to be toric, with the anterior corneal astigmatism apparently correcting astigmatism due to other ocular refracting surfaces. Will residual astigmatism be present in this case if a soft contact lens is worn?

84. toric (or spherocylindrical)

85. You will remember that, by convention, the meridians of an ophthalmic lens are numbered 0 to 180 degrees, with 0 degrees at the 3 o'clock position and counterclockwise progression to 180 degrees when the lens is viewed from the front. On the diagram the unnumbered heavy line indicates the _____ degrees meridian of the lens.

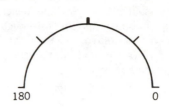

180   0

---

256. 1.25

257. Complete absence of accommodation does not occur with any cycloplegic. There is thus always some measurable _____ accommodation following a cycloplegic drug.

---

428. near

429. The near P.D., determined as described, measures the distance between the visual axes in the plane of the ruler. This is desirable, since this is the approximate plane in which lenses will be placed.

    The near P.D. is a measurement of the distance between the (1) _____ while the patient fixates at 14 inches. The plane of P.D. measurement is located (2) (in/in front of/behind) the plane of the trial and prescribed lenses.

600. (*Advance to next frame.*)

---

601. A single image is perceived if each eye is fixating on the same object with the fovea and the eyes have the usual retinal correspondence. This ability to see an object as one (although both retinas are used simultaneously) is called fusion. The perception of two retinal images (one in each eye) as a single image is called _____ .

---

772. 5.00

---

773. A patient whose working distance is 25 cm has an amplitude of accommodation of 5.00 D. He will require an add of 1.50 D to read comfortably at this point. (He can use 2.50 D of accommodation, so he needs 1.50 to give him the 4.00 D necessary for 25 cm and still have 50 percent of his accommodation in reserve.) At 33.33 cm, another patient's working distance, this patient can read print through −1.00 D spheres OU added to his distance correction, but −1.25 D blurs the print. He has (1) _____ D accommodation and thus can use (2) _____ D at his working distance and still keep one half in reserve. Therefore, he will need an add (additional plus) of (3) _____ D for a working distance of 33.33 cm.

---

944. No

---

945. Residual astigmatism can be predicted by comparing the spectacle refraction with the measurements of the radii of curvature of the cornea. One instrument which measures the radii of curvature of the anterior corneal surface is called a Keratometer. The _____ readings can be compared with spectacle refraction to predict the presence of residual astigmatism.

85. 90

---

86. On a toric surface there is a meridian of least power and a meridian of most power. These meridians are designated in degrees on an ophthalmic lens with 0 degrees on your (1) _____ and 180 degrees on your (2) _____ as the lens faces you.

---

257. residual

---

258. The effectiveness of a cycloplegic drug is assessed by determining the minimal residual accommodation obtainable with full dosage of a given concentration of the drug. A cycloplegic which results in a residual accommodation of more than 2.00 D is not considered adequate for refraction. To be useful in refraction, a cycloplegic must result in no more than (1) _____ D of (2) _____.

---

429. (1) visual axes
    (2) in

430.
  The diagram measures the (near/distant) P.D.

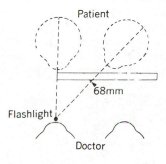

601. fusion

---

602. Only if both retinal images are fused into a single image can the third dimension be perceived. In most instances the two retinal images are quite similar, differing only in the slight angle of viewing caused by the separation of the two eyes. These slight differences in the two retinal images give clues as to depth (depth perception).

A prerequisite for depth perception is (1) _____ of the slightly different images. These differences are caused by (2) _____.

---

773. (1) 4.00
    (2) 2.00
    (3) 1.00

---

774. The near point of accommodation, measured binocularly with the distance correction in place, is the nearest point to the eye at which the patient can see small print clearly. This distance converted to diopters is the amplitude of accommodation.

If the print blurs at 12.5 cm, the near point of accommodation is (1) _____ and the amplitude of accommodation is (2) _____.

---

945. Keratometer

---

946. Keratometry utilizes the property of the anterior surface of the cornea to act as a small convex mirror. The instrument measures the size of a reflected image, and the image size varies with the radius of curvature of the corneal mirror. Measurements of the radii of curvature of the anterior surface of the cornea are made by a (1) _____ utilizing the (2) _____ of an image reflected from the corneal surface.

86. (1) right
(2) left

---

87. If there are two curves ground on the spherical surface of a meniscus lens, a type of bifocal lens called a **one piece bifocal** is created. The difference in power between the two areas of the lens is termed the **add.** The add in each of these bifocals is _____ D.

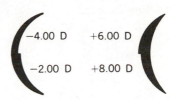

−4.00 D +6.00 D

−2.00 D +8.00 D

---

258. (1) 2.00
(2) residual accommodation

---

259. Mydriasis accompanies cycloplegia, but the degree of mydriasis is unrelated to the degree of cycloplegia. Despite the degree of pupillary dilation, the effectivity of cycloplegic can only be determined by measuring _____ .

---

430. near

---

431. To measure the distance P.D., proceed as if to measure the near P.D. with your OS opposite the patient's OD, the flashlight held close to your OS, and the zero on the ruler aligned with the corneal reflex OD. Move the flashlight to just below your OD, close your OS, and read the distance P.D. on the millimeter rule by noting the position of the corneal reflex in the patient's OS as the patient continues to look at the flashlight.

To measure the distance P.D., begin as if to measure near P.D., then move the flashlight to a point near your (1) _____ , close your (2) _____ , and read the ruler noting the position of the corneal reflex in the patient's (3) _____ .

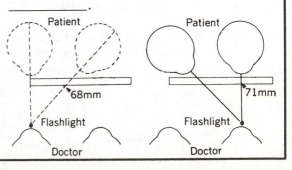

602. (1) fusion

(2) separation of the two eyes giving different views (or similar wording)

---

603. The perception of the third dimension allows us to appreciate relative depth. The sense of the third dimension is called _____.

---

774. (1) 12.5 cm

(2) 8.00 D

---

775. If the near point of accommodation is 12.5 cm, the amplitude of accommodation is (1) _____ D, and (2) _____ D add is necessary for a working distance of 20 cm (keeping one-half of the accommodation in reserve).

---

946. (1) Keratometer

(2) size (or magnification)

---

947. Keratometer readings may be expressed in diopters of refractive power if suitable allowance is made for the index of refraction of the cornea. The instruments themselves have been calibrated for this purpose and tables are available which may also be used. Keratometry readings are usually expressed in _____.

87. 2.00

88. A difference in spherical power between two areas of a lens may also be created by fusing into a depression of variable curvature a button of glass with a higher index of refraction than the main lens. A bifocal manufactured in this manner is termed a **fused bifocal,** and the fused segment is on the front of a meniscus lens. The curve of the front of the segment is continuous with, and the same as, the front curve of the rest of the lens. The add in a fused bifocal (can/cannot) be determined from measurements of surface curvatures.

259. residual accommodation

260. The ideal cycloplegic for refraction results in fast, complete, safe cycloplegia with rapid recovery. Drug A produces the same degree of cycloplegia as drug B at the same time and both are equally safe. Recovery from the effect of drug A takes four days and from the effect of drug B two days. Which drug comes closer to the ideal cycloplegic for refraction?

431. (1) OD
　　(2) OS
　　(3) OS

432. The diagram depicts a P.D. of (1) _____ mm at near and (2) _____ mm at distance.

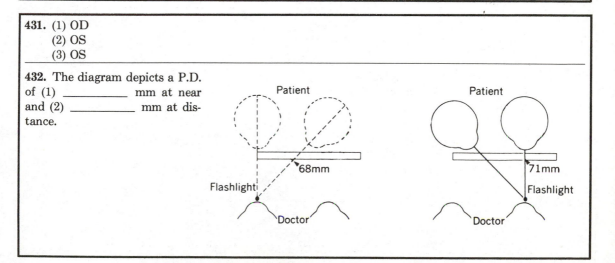

603. depth perception (or steropsis)

---

604. The ability to fuse two retinal images (one in each eye) into one and to perceive depth is regarded as Grade III fusion. A lesser amount of fusion (Grade II) consists of perceiving one image from the two retinal images with fusional reserve. In Grade II fusion the eyes can be made to diverge or converge and still utilize both foveal images and perceive one, but without depth perception.

Grade III fusion means the patient has

_____.

---

775. (1) 8.00
(2) 1.00

---

776. The two basic methods of measuring the amplitude of accommodation are:

(a) Measure the amount of minus through which a patient can still see clearly (at any known distance).

(b) Note the nearest point (the near point) at which the patient can see clearly.

Method (a) consists of measuring the amplitude of accommodation with (1) _____ lenses.

Method (b) consists of pushing the reading material toward the patient until the print starts to (2) _____ .

---

947. diopters

---

948. Keratometry readings of a patient's cornea are 42.75 D in all meridians. The patient's corneal surface is (spherical/toric).

88. cannot

---

89. If a bifocal lens must have a toric surface, the toric surface is ground on the side opposite the segment. In a fused bifocal the toric surface will be on the (anterior/posterior) side.

---

260. B

---

261. Of the cycloplegic drugs in common use, atropine is the most effective and homatropine the least. Cyclopentolate, tropicamide, and scopolamine are all more effective than homatropine. If, as in refracting a patient with strabismus, maximum cycloplegia is desired, what is the drug of choice?

---

432. (1) 68
(2) 71

---

433. The diagrammed P.D. measures _____ mm.

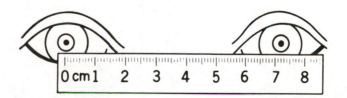

604. depth perception (or steropsis)

---

605. Grade I fusion means only that the patient can perceive two dissimilar retinal images as a single image without fusional reserve or depth perception. If the right eye sees Figure A and the left eye sees Figure B, a patient with Grade I fusion would see these Grade I targets as (*sketch your answer*).

A   B

---

776. (1) minus
     (2) blur

---

777. Cross cylinders may be used to determine the necessary bifocal add by creating a conoid of Sturm. Place the target—a printed grid—at the desired working distance. Place 0.50 D cross cylinders (OU) with minus axis at 90 degrees, creating an astigmatism (remember that a cylinder focuses lines parallel to the cylinder's axis) before both eyes which have been corrected and balanced for distance. If the patient has no accommodation the entire conoid will be behind the retina but he will see the _____ lines blackest since they are parallel to the plus axis of the cross cylinder, and hence nearer to the retina.

Target

---

948. spherical

---

949. Keratometer readings of a cornea are 42.75 D in the 180 degree meridian and 41.75 D in the 90 degree meridian. This corneal surface is (1) _____ and the eye has anterior corneal (2) _____ .

89. posterior

---

90. A lens without a bifocal is termed a single vision lens. The weaker curve of a single vision lens without a cylinder is termed the _____ curve.

---

261. Atropine

---

262. *(See Table 1, p. 354.)* Which of the listed drugs has the longest duration of maximum cycloplegia?

---

433. 71 (or 72)

---

434. A trial frame is a device for holding trial lenses in proper position during refraction and must allow fitting adjustments for the facial contour of patients and also positioning adjustments for the lenses. The adjustable features of a trial frame allow for variation in (1) _____ and (2) _____ .

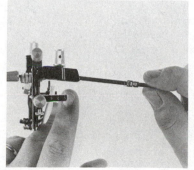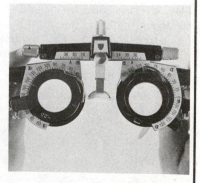

605.

606. Grade I fusion means that the patient has simultaneous macular perception. If patient sees Figure A (Grade I target) with OD and sees Figure B (Grade I target) with OS, sketch what he will see with Grade I fusion.

A   **B**

---

777. horizontal

778. With the cross cylinders in place OU and the grid target at the patient's usual working distance, add equal plus OU until the patient reports the vertical lines are blacker. Then reduce plus until both vertical and horizontal lines are reported to be equally black.

Plus lenses are increased until the (1) _____ are blacker, then reduced until (2) _____.

---

949. (1) toric
(2) astigmatism

950. A cornea measures 44.00 D curvature in the 90 degree meridian and 42.00 D curvature in the 180 degree meridian. This astigmatism would be corrected by a spectacle lens with a −2.00 D cylinder at axis _____.

90. base

---

91. The base curve of a single vision meniscus lens with a toric surface is the weaker powered curve on the toric surface. In this lens, the base curve is _____ D.

+6.00 D →
+8.00 D →
−2.00 D

---

262. Atropine

---

263. *(See Table 1.)* Which of the drugs has the longest recovery time until accommodation is normal?

---

434. (1) facial contour ⎫ either
(2) positioning of lenses ⎭ order

---

435. A trial frame properly adjusted aligns the optical centers of the trial lenses with the visual axis of each eye, with the lenses perpendicular to the direction of gaze. During refraction the optical centers of the trial lenses should be aligned with the _____ of each eye.

606.

607. If a patient can fuse Grade I targets at a point from 10Δ (Δ = prism diopters) base in (in front of his eyes) to 10Δ base out (in front of his eyes) we would say he has 10Δ B.I. and 10Δ B.O. fusional reserve.

He has at least Grade _____ fusion. (Grade I fusion and fusional reserve = Grade II fusion.)

---

778. (1) vertical lines
(2) both horizontal and vertical lines are equally black

779. The cross cylinder test is useful for determining the add at the working distance. The cross grid in the test is placed at _____.

---

950. 180 degrees

951. Keratometry readings (K readings) of a given cornea are 44.00 D at 90 degrees and 42.00 D at 180 degrees. The spectacle correction is $-2.00 \; -2.00 \times 180$. Residual astigmatism (is/is not) expected.

91. $+6.00$

---

92. The base curve of a meniscus bifocal is the curve ground on the segment side of the lens. In a fused bifocal the segment is on the front of the lens. The base curve of a fused meniscus bifocal is the _____ surface.

---

263. Atropine

---

264. *(See Table 1.)* Which drug is usually instilled 6 to 8 times at intervals of 10 to 15 minutes?

---

435. visual axis

---

436. Facial contours of the brow, distance between eyes, distance from eyes to ears, and bridge of the nose vary and affect the fit of the spectacles; hence, adjustable parts of a trial frame must number at least _____ for fitting purposes.

607. II

---

608. One instrument used to view fusion targets and to move them is called a synoptophore.

An instrument to present targets and measure fusional amplitude is called a(n) _____ .

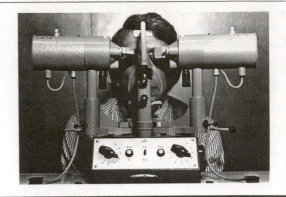

---

779. the usual near working distance

---

780. The astigmatic correction must be in place before the cross cylinder test can be used to determine the add. If too much minus cylinder at axis 90 degrees has been prescribed in the distance correction, the _____ lines on the grid will be blacker (without accommodation) before the cross cylinder is in position.

---

951. is not

---

952. K readings are 44.00 D at 90 degrees and 42.00 D at 180 degrees. The spectacle correction is −2.00 −.50 × 90. Residual astigmatism is expected and will be _____ D.

92. convex (or front)

---

93. Examine the drawing of the Geneva lens gauge. This instrument has three prongs at its foot, the outer two fixed and the central one movable. When the gauge is held against a flat surface, as in the drawing, the indicator points to _____ D power.

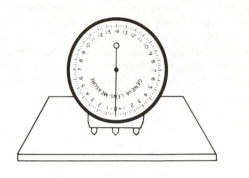

---

264. Homatropine

---

265. *(See Table 1.)* How soon after instillation of the second drop is cycloplegia maximum with cyclopentolate?

---

436. four

---

437. The distance from eye to ear is termed temple length. Examine the trial frame and note that the _____ can be varied by sliding the earpiece forward and backward.

608. synoptophore

---

609. If the two eyes cannot bring images together into a single image, we may have diplopia (double vision). Diplopia is frequently produced as a means of testing certain parameters of binocular vision. If we place more prism diopters in front of a patient than he has fusional reserve, he may report

_____ .

---

780. horizontal

---

781. After a tentative add has been selected the range of clear vision at near should be ascertained. This is measured by moving the print toward the patient until blurring occurs and then away from the patient until blurring occurs.

An add has been calculated for a patient with a working distance of 16 inches. Print can be read until it is brought to 10 inches from the eyes and until it is taken to 26 inches from the eyes. The range of clear vision is from (1) _____ to (2) _____ .

---

952. 2.50

---

953. Spectacle correction is −3.50. K readings are 41.00 D at 90 degrees and 42.50 D at 180 degrees. Residual astigmatism of (1) _____ D
$\overline{\text{(sign and power)}}$
at axis (2) _____ degrees is expected when the hard contact lens is in place.

186

93. zero

94. The lens gauge measures the radius of curvature of a surface. The dial is calibrated in diopters from -20 to $+20$. The radius of curvature of a lens surface can be converted to dioptric power only if the index of refraction of the lens is known. The lens gauge is calibrated for a glass of a specific index of refraction, usually crown glass with an index of refraction of 1.523. The lens gauge cannot give accurate readings in diopters of curvature for each of two lenses of different _____.

265. 25 minutes

266. *(See Table 1.)* How soon after using homatropine is a patient's accommodation sufficient for reading?

437. temple length

438. You will remember that the interpupillary distance, or P.D., is expressed in millimeters. The ruled area on the front of the horizontal bar of the trial frame is calibrated in millimeters and is used to conform to the _____.

609. diplopia

---

610. Fusion can be interrupted by presenting a totally different target to each eye. When fusion is interrupted the eyes are said to be dissociated. The absence of fusion implies _____ of the eyes.

---

781. (1) 10 inches ⎱ either
     (2) 26 inches ⎰ order

---

782. In patients wearing near corrections the range of clear vision anterior to the working distance should equal dioptrically the range behind the working distance. (This is another way of stating that 50 percent of accommodation should be in reserve.) The ranges anterior and posterior to the working distance should be equal in (diopters/inches) when a patient wears the appropriate near correction.

---

953. (1) −1.50   or   (1) +1.50
     (2) 90   (2) 180

---

954. Only K readings along the visual axis are useful in predicting residual astigmatism since the power of the cornea decreases markedly away from the apex. K readings in the corneal periphery (can/cannot) be used to predict residual astigmatism.

94. indices of refraction.

95. The drawing shows a convex surface being measured with the Geneva lens gauge. The indicator points to _____ .
(sign and power)

---

266. 6 hours

267. *(See Table 1.)* The drug with the fastest onset and shortest duration of maximum effect is _____ .

---

438. P.D. (or interpupillary distance)

439. The lens-carrying part of the trial frame can be moved horizontally for each eye separately by turning the uppermost small wheels at the outermost ends of the horizontal bar. Turn these wheels on any available trial frame and note the movement of the lens-carrying portion of the trial frame, permitting variation in the _____ .

610. dissociation

---

611. The tendency to see singly is great, so to examine the properties of binocular vision some method for dissociation is necessary. One method of dissociation is to have one eye see a line, the other a dot of light. The eyes will be dissociated because the line and dot are _____ targets.

---

782. diopters

---

783. A patient, wearing the appropriate near correction has clear vision from his working distance of 13 inches (3.00 D) to 10 inches (4.00 D)—a difference of 1.00 D. He can see the print until it is 20 inches (2.00 D) from his eyes. (3.00 D − 1.00 D = 2.00 D).

A patient, wearing a near correction, has clear vision from his working distance at 16 inches (2.50 D) to 10 inches (4.00 D)—a difference of 1.50 D. Moving the print away, he should be able to see clearly until it is _____ inches from his eyes.

---

954. cannot

---

955. Since the power of the anterior corneal periphery is much less than the power at the apex, hard contact lenses are designed with peripheral posterior radii of curvature (greater than/ less than) the central posterior radius of curvature.

95. +6.50 D

96. The drawing shows the measurement of a concave surface. This is the concave side of the lens. The convex surface measured +6.50 D in the previous frame. The approximate total power of this lens as derived from the algebraic sum of the two surface powers is _____.

(sign and power)

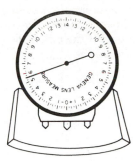

267. tropicamide

268. *(See Table 1.)* List the drugs in order of increasing duration of maximum effect.

439. P.D. (or interpupillary distance)

440. As the lens-carrying part of the frame is moved horizontally, the vertical line at the top of this part of the frame passes beneath the ruled area of the horizontal bar. This ruled area is a measure of the center of the lens carrier of each eye from the midline. The sum of the distances of the center of each lens from the midline should equal the P.D. If the P.D. is 62 mm, the lens carrier of the trial frame will be set at _____ before each eye.

611. dissimilar

612. A horizontal deviation of dissociated eyes can be measured with the appropriate base in or base out prism. When the patient sees a dot with one eye and a vertical line with the other, the correct prism will align the dot on the _____ .

783. 40

784. If a presbyopic patient is a hyperope who has never worn glasses, correcting his hyperopia may suffice for near as well as distance. If a 1.50 D OU hyperope, age 40, has presbyopic symptoms, a prescription of +1.50 D OU to correct his hyperopia will allow him to see clearly and comfortably (50 percent of accommodation in reserve) to a near working distance of _____ cm.

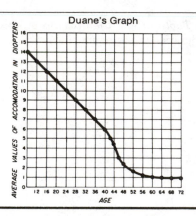

Duane's Graph

955. greater than

956. Peripheral posterior curves of a hard contact lens are made flatter than the central posterior curve. This is because _____ .

96. +1.00 D

---

97. The base curve of the lens just measured is
_____ D.

- Concave side = −5.50 D.
- Convex side = +6.50 D.

---

268. Tropicamide, cyclopentolate and homatropine, scopolamine, atropine (either order for second and third)

---

269. *(See Table 1.)* List the drugs in order of increasing time of onset of maximum effect.

---

440. 31

---

441. For purposes of proper adjustment of a trial frame, a patient's P.D. has been measured. The measurement so found must be divided by _____ before the lens carriers can be set according to the calibration on the horizontal bar.

612. line (vertical line)

613. If a light is viewed through a glass rod, a streak of light is seen perpendicular to the length of the rod. The reason for this is that this rod is a high-powered cylindrical lens and the line parallel to the rod is focused just behind it—about 10 mm or less from the eye—so the eye would require 1000/10 or at least 100 D of power to focus it. The other meridian not affected by the lens would be seen as a streak. The image of light seen through a rod is a streak _____ to the rod.

784. 33.33

785. The needed power of the add at near determines whether or not bifocals should be suggested to the patient rather than only the distance correction. In general, if the needed add is less than +1.25 D, wait until a greater need arises before prescribing bifocals. In general, do not prescribe bifocals with adds less than _____ D.

956. the periphery of the cornea is flatter than the apex (or similar wording)

957. Hard contact lenses may be ground with a toric anterior surface, a toric posterior surface, or both. Toric hard contact lenses could be used to fit corneas with high astigmatic error or to correct residual astigmatism. Astigmatic contact lens problems can be resolved by using _____ hard contact lenses.

97. −5.50

---

98. Cylinders can be measured with a lens gauge. As the gauge is rotated on a cylindrical surface the difference between the greatest and smallest readings indicates the cylindrical power. The drawing shows the maximum measurement of a convex surface. This is_____ and represents
(sign and power)
the power of one of the principal meridians.

---

269. Tropicamide, cyclopentolate, homatropine, scopolamine, atropine

---

270. A drug which results in a residual accommodation greater than _____ is unsatisfactory for refraction.

---

441. two

---

442. The position of the nosepiece can be varied vertically and anteroposteriorly by turning the wheels in the center of the horizontal bar. Turn the wheels in the center of the horizontal bar. The wheel directly at the top of this bar and perpendicular to it controls the _____ movements of the nosepiece.

613. perpendicular

---

614. The Maddox rod is a series of rods or grooves and functions just as a single rod, giving a linear image of a spot of light. The image is _____ to the axis of the rods.

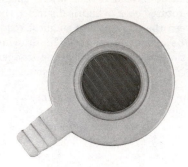

---

785. + 1.25

---

786. The Franklin bifocal was the first bifocal. This was composed of two lenses cut in half with the upper portion for distance and the lower for near. (1) (A/B) is the distance portion and (2) (A/B) has more plus power.

---

957. toric

---

958. Despite the ability to create toric hard contact lenses, this is seldom done in practice because of fitting problems. Almost all hard contact lenses prescribed are therefore _____.

98. +10.00 D

---

99. The drawing shows the lens surface that was in the previous frame being measured. Now the lens gauge has been turned 90 degrees, and the other principal meridian is being measured. This meridian measures (1) _____ ; thus the cylinder

(sign and power)
is (2)_____ D. (The other meridian mea-

(power)
sured +10.00 D.)

---

270. 2.00 D

---

271. Of the drugs previously listed, the least residual accommodation occurs with use of (1) _____ and the most residual accommodation occurs with use of (2) _____ .

---

442. vertical

---

443. The pantoscopic tilt of a spectacle frame refers to the angle the lens makes with the temple. This tilt is varied to maintain the lens perpendicular to the direction of gaze and to allow for variation in brow prominence. Brow prominence can be compensated for in the fitting of spectacles by variation of the _____ .

614. perpendicular

---

615. The Maddox rod serves well as a means of dissociating the eyes. If you place a Maddox rod (frequently tinted red) in front of the right eye (with the rods horizontal) while having the patient view a small light at a distance the image on the retinas will be: (*See figure at right.*)

    If the patient has Grade I fusion, he will see both (1) _____ and (2) _____.

White light —● |— Red streak

OS   OD

---

786. (1) A
    (2) B

---

787. The segment of a bifocal has more plus power than the distance portion of the lens to enable the presbyope to see clearly at near. This additional plus power is termed the add. The plus necessary for the presbyope to see clearly at near is called the

_____.

---

958. spherical

---

959. The effective power of minus lenses (increases/decreases) when the vertex distance of the lens is decreased.

99. (1) +8.25 D
   (2) 1.75

---

100. The drawing again shows the 180 degree meridian being measured. (The 90 degree meridian measured +10.00 D.) The base curve (the weaker curve of this toric surface) is _____ D.

---

271. (1) atropine
   (2) homatropine

---

272. *(See Table 1.)* Cyclopentolate and tropicamide are usually instilled (1) _____ times at intervals of (2) _____ .

---

443. pantoscopic tilt

---

444. The pantoscopic tilt can be seen when a trial frame or spectacles are viewed from the side. View the trial frame from the side, turn the wheel projecting upward from either temple, and note the variation of the _____ of the frame.

615. (1) the light   either

      (2) the red streak   order

616. With the Maddox rod in front of the right eye the patient's eyes are dissociated. If he has at least Grade I fusion and his visual axes remain aligned with the target he will see which image? (A/B/C).

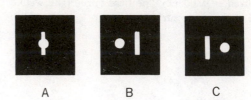

A   B   C

---

787. add

788. The Franklin bifocal was composed of two lenses cut through the optical centers and cemented together with the optical centers adjoining. At the optical center of a lens there is (1) _____ prismatic power, so there (2) (is/is no) prismatic power change as the visual axis moves from the lower portion of the distance lens to the upper portion of the near lens.

---

959. increases

960. An eye corrected by a -12.00 D lens, vertex distance 11 mm, will be corrected by a contact lens of approximately _____ D.

100. +8.25

---

101. The drawing shows the concave surface of a single vision lens being measured. This reading remains the same as the lens gauge is rotated. The approximate total power in the 90 degree meridian is (1) _____ D, and in the 180 degree
(sign and power)
meridian it is (2) _____ D. (The other
(sign and power)
side measured +10.00 D at 90 degrees and +8.25 D at 180 degrees.)

---

272. (1) two
(2) five minutes

---

273. *(See Table 1.)* Atropine ointment is usually instilled (1) _____ daily for (2) _____ days prior to refraction.

---

444. pantoscopic tilt

---

445. Adjustment of (1) _____, (2) _____, (3) _____ and (4) _____ can be made to make the trial frame conform to the patient's facial contour.

616. A

---

617. If the patient's dissociated eye remains on line with the target, he is orthophoric (or said to have orthophoria). The absence of orthophoria is termed heterophoria. Using a Maddox rod to dissociate the eye the illustrated image would represent _____ .

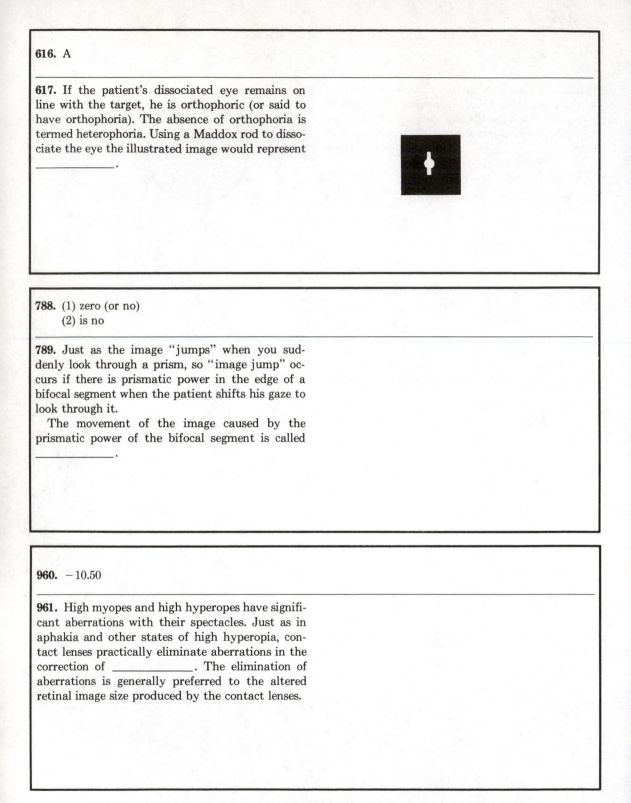

---

788. (1) zero (or no)
  (2) is no

---

789. Just as the image "jumps" when you suddenly look through a prism, so "image jump" occurs if there is prismatic power in the edge of a bifocal segment when the patient shifts his gaze to look through it.

  The movement of the image caused by the prismatic power of the bifocal segment is called

_____ .

---

960. − 10.50

---

961. High myopes and high hyperopes have significant aberrations with their spectacles. Just as in aphakia and other states of high hyperopia, contact lenses practically eliminate aberrations in the correction of _____ . The elimination of aberrations is generally preferred to the altered retinal image size produced by the contact lenses.

101. (1) +3.50
(2) +1.75

---

102. The formula of the lens just previously shown being measured may be written as a combination of sphere and plus cylinder as +1.75 D sphere combined with +1.75 D cylinder axis _____ degrees. (The axis of a cylinder is 90 degrees from the measurable surface power.) The lens measured −6.50 D on the concave surface, +8.25 D in the 180 degree meridian, and +10.00 D in the 90 degree meridian on the convex surface.

---

273. (1) one time
(2) three

---

274. *(See Table 1.)* Full recovery of accommodation following atropine requires _____.

---

445. (1) temple length   (3) pantoscopic tilt ⎫ any
(2) P.D. (or interpupillary distance)   (4) nosepiece ⎭ order

---

446. The lens carrier of the trial frame consists of four cells for holding trial lenses, each lens held in position by a spring clip. Examine the frame. The front surface of the lens carrier has (1) _____ cell(s) and the back surface (2) _____ cell(s).

617. orthophoria

618. If one eye deviates nasally, the image will fall on the nasal side of the retina (patient will interpret nasal stimuli as being in the temporal field). The patient will have uncrossed diplopia. The right eye projects its image to which side of the image of the left eye when either eye deviates nasally? (Right/Left).

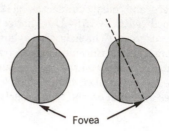

Fovea

789. image jump

790. Since the Franklin bifocal is composed of two lenses cut through their optical centers and joined there, an image jump (occurs/does not occur) as the patient's gaze shifts from the distance to the bifocal segment.

961. high myopia

962. In high plus and minus refractive errors, contact lenses are usually optically superior to spectacles because they eliminate many _____.

102. 180

---

103. The symbol, $\subset$, is used to indicate "combined with," and the symbol, $\times$, is used to represent "axis." C stands for cylinder, and S for sphere. A symbol for degrees is omitted. The formula of a spherocylindrical lens may be written $+1.50$ S $\subset$ $+2.00$ C $\times$ 90. Using the standard symbols, write the formula of a $+6.00$ D sphere combined with a $+2.00$ D cylinder at axis 135 degrees.

---

274. 10 to 14 days

---

275. *(See Table 1.)* How soon after the use of atropine is a patient able to read?

---

446. (1) three
　　　(2) one

---

447. When lenses are placed into a trial frame, the strongest spherical lens is placed in the back cell of the frame. With a combination of trial lenses measuring $+2.00$ D sphere, $+0.25$ D sphere, and -0.75 D cylinder, the lens in the back cell of the trial frame will be _____.

618. Right

---

619. If we have a Maddox rod in front of a right eye which deviates nasally when dissociated, the patient will see (A/B/C).

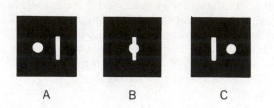

A   B   C

---

790. does not occur

---

791. The dividing line between the distance and near portions of the Franklin bifocal was cosmetically objectionable. An early improvement was the wafer biocal which was cemented on the posterior surface of the lens. One advantage of the wafer bifocal is the easy manner in which the add can be changed. In conditions which require temporary bifocals, the _____ bifocal is ideal.

---

962. aberrations

---

963. Contact lenses are indicated for the correction of (1) _____ and (2)
<u>(type of refractive error)</u>
_____ . They are less successful
<u>(type of refractive error)</u>
in the correction of (3) _____ .
<u>(type of refractive error)</u>

103. $+6.00$ S $\frown$ $+2.00$ C $\times$ 135

---

104. In practice the symbols S, $\frown$, and C, may be omitted when lens formulae are written. The formula for a lens may read $+1.50$ $+2.00$ $\times$ 90. Rewrite the formula inserting the symbols S, $\frown$, and C, in the appropriate places.

---

275. Three to four days

---

276. *(See Table 1.)* How soon after cyclopentolate is a patient able to read?

---

447. $+2.00$ D sphere

---

448. The front surface of the lens carrier is calibrated in degrees from 0 to 180 in a _____ direction, conforming with the designation of meridians of an ophthalmic lens.

619. A

---

620. When the eye's position of rest, after dissociation, is nasally, we call the condition esophoria. If the patient reports uncrossed diplopia after dissociation, he has _____.

---

791. wafer type

---

792. A disadvantage of any cement type bifocal is the tendency for the cement to crack when sudden temperature changes are encountered. Wafer bifocals (are/are not) indicated in a butcher who goes in and out of a cold room.

---

963. (1) high hyperopia (aphakia) ⎱ either
     (2) high myopia   ⎰ order
     (3) high astigmatic errors

---

964. Vision in irregular corneal astigmatism and keratoconus may be improved by hard contact lenses when spectacles prove inadequate. Hard contact lenses may be superior to spectacles to correct vision in (1) _____ and in (2) _____.

104. $+1.50\ \text{S} \subset +2.00\ \text{C} \times 90$

---

105. $+3.00 \subset -1.00 \times 180$ indicates that a $+3.00$ D sphere is combined with a cylinder of -1.00 D $\times$ 180. The symbol $\subset$ means combined with.

Minus 4.00 D sphere combined with a minus cylinder of 2.00 D the axis of which is 90 degrees is written _____ .

---

276. Three hours

---

277. A practical method of obtaining cycloplegia comparable to the use of atropine consists of first instilling proparacaine 0.5 percent followed in 10 seconds by successive drops of cyclopentolate 2 percent and tropicamide 1 percent. The proparacaine not only increases the penetration of the cycloplegics but prevents the discomfort usually associated with their instillation. How soon should the above combination have its maximum effect? *(See Table 1.)*

---

448. counterclockwise

---

449. Turning the wheel at the outer side of each carrier results in rotation of the (anterior/posterior) cell(s).

620. esophoria

---

621. If the dissociated eye deviates temporally, the image will fall on the temporal side of the retina (which will be interpreted as being nasal), and crossed diplopia will be reported. If the right eye deviates temporally, it projects its image to which side of the image of the left eye?

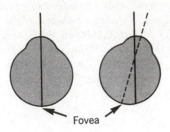

Fovea

---

792. are not

---

793. About the only use of the wafer bifocal today is in accommodative esotropia (the turning in of the eyes at near due to overaccommodation and hence overconvergence) where temporary bifocals are frequently tried. The wafer bifocals are inexpensive and easily positioned by an optician.

The suitable type bifocal for an accommodative esotropia is _____.

---

964. (1) irregular corneal astigmatism
(2) keratoconus } either order

---

965. Since the successful fitting of bifocal contact lenses is relatively difficult, contact lenses usually are not indicated for the correction of _____.

105. $-4.00 \mathbin{\bigcirc} -2.00 \times 90$

---

106. A -8.00 D lens combined with a $+6.00$ D cylinder the axis of which is 120 degrees is written

_____.

If you wish, you may omit the symbol $\bigcirc$.

---

277. 25 minutes (the time of the slower drug)

---

278. The subjective tests for measurement of residual accommodation do not eliminate the effect of depth of focus. This is estimated to account for about 1.00 D of the residual accommodation found with these tests. The allowable residual accommodation for refraction following a cycloplegic is (1) _____ of which 1.00 D may be the result of (2) _____.

---

449. anterior

---

450. Phoropters are often used instead of trial frames and loose lenses. A phoropter contains spherical, cylindrical, and diagnostic lenses mounted in wheels. Rotation of the wheels accomplishes change in power of the lenses before the eye. The patient places his head against the perfectly leveled instrument. Since movement of the head may alter the direction of the visual axis, a head rest should be positioned behind the patient to minimize head movement. A phoropter, therefore, should always be used with a _____ in order to keep the visual axis aligned with the lenses.

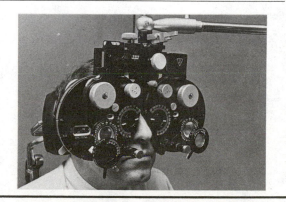

621. Left

---

622. The turning temporally of a dissociated eye is termed exophoria. Crossed diplopia, as reported by a patient after dissociation, implies he has

_____ .

---

793. the wafer (bifocal)

---

794. The anterior surface of the wafer segment is spherical and conforms to the posterior lens surface. Thus, any cylinder in the lens will have to be ground on the _____ surface of the lens to insure a good fit of the add.

---

965. presbyopia

966.

PART XIII

APHAKIA

(Advance to next frame.)

106. $-8.00 + 6.00 \times 120$

---

107. The power of a cylinder is 90 degrees away from the axis. Consider the lens -3.00 S $+5.00$ C $\times$ 60. This means that at 150 degrees (90 degrees away from 60 degrees) the power of the lens is the sum of -3.00 D and $+5.00$ D or (1) _____ D.

At its axis a cylinder has no power, so at 60 degrees the power of the lens -3.00 S $+5.00$ C $\times$ 60 is (2) _____ D.

---

278. (1) 2.00 D
(2) depth of focus

---

279. Instillation of homatropine may be followed by temporary stimulation of accommodation prior to the onset of cycloplegia. It is therefore particularly important to measure _____ when refracting with homatropine.

---

450. headrest

---

451. Just as with trial frames, the P.D. of phoropters is adjustable. When using a phoropter, the (1) _____ must be adjusted and a (2) _____ used to keep the visual axes aligned with the lens centers.

622. exophoria

---

623. After dissociation with a Maddox rod OD, the patient with exophoria reports (A/B/C).

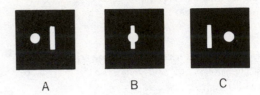

A   B   C

---

794. anterior

---

795. The Kryptok bifocal was the first fused bifocal and remains a practical, inexpensive bifocal. It consists of a segment of flint glass fused into a countersink in the anterior surface of a crown glass lens.

This diagrams the production of a _____ fused bifocal.

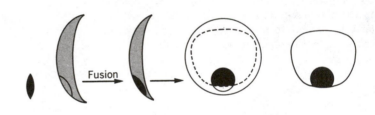

Fusion

---

966. (*Advance to next frame.*)

---

967. Removal of the crystalline lens from the eye results in a(n) (1) (increase/decrease) in the total refracting power of the eye. In most patients, therefore, the eye becomes highly (2)

_____
(type of refractive error).

107. (1) $+2.00$
    (2) -3.00

---

108. Remember:

sphere   cylinder

$-8.00 \; \frown \; +6.00 \times 120$ indicates that the power at 120 degrees is (1) _____ D and the power at 30 degrees is (2) _____ D.

---

279. (residual) accommodation

---

280. Sympathomimetic drugs, such as epinephrine, cocaine, and neosynephrine, have little or no cycloplegic effect. The group of drugs classed as _____ is not suitable for cycloplegic refractions.

---

451. (1) P.D. (or interpupillary distance)
    (2) headrest

---

452. The main advantage of a phoropter is that lens powers may be changed rapidly as compared with a trial frame and loose lenses. The disadvantages of a phoropter are that young children may be frightened by it, that it is hard to see the patient's eyes through it, and that the distance between the eye and lenses (vertex distance) is greater than in eyeglasses. As will be shown later, the vertex distance is of major importance in prescribing high plus and high minus lenses. For the reasons given it is necessary at times to refract using a _____ rather than a phoropter.

623. C

---

624. The deviations of the dissociated eye nasally or temporally are termed horizontal phorias. Vertical phorias do exist and should be checked. Rotation of the dissociating Maddox rod to the vertical position permits this measurement and causes the patient to see a horizontal line. In the absence of vertical phoria (vertical orthophoria) the patient sees (A/B/C).

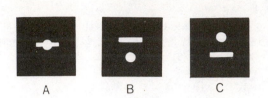

A   B   C

---

795. Kryptok

---

796. You will recall that:

Prism diopters = decentration (in cm) × power (in diopters).

This is called Prentice's rule and is used to determine prismatic effect at any point in a lens.

At a point 4 mm (0.4 cm) below the optical center of a −7.50 D lens there will be a prismatic effect of (1) _____ base (2) _____ .

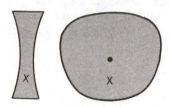

---

967. (1) decrease
(2) hyperopic (or hypermetropic)

---

968. The crystalline lens has an average power of +20.00 D. A spectacle lens used to replace the crystalline lens of the eye is positioned well anterior to the cornea and hence will be (stronger/weaker) then +20.00 D.

108. (1) -8.00
  (2) -2.00

---

109. If there is $+6.00$ D power at 90 degrees and $+8.00$ D power at 180 degrees, then a 2.00 D cylinder exists. This could be a -2.00 D cylinder axis 180 degrees or a $+2.00$ D cylinder axis _____ degrees.

---

280. sympathomimetic

---

281. Atropine or the combination of proparacaine, cyclopentolate, and tropicamide are the cycloplegics of choice any time there is a question of a strabismus and for most refractions in preschool children. The atropine should be given (1) _____ time(s) per day for (2) _____ day(s) prior to refraction.

---

452. trial frame (and loose lenses)

453.

PART VI

RETINOSCOPY

(Advance to next frame.)

624. A

---

625. You will recall that 1Δ (prism diopter) deviates parallel rays of light 1 cm at 1 m behind the prism.

We can convert prism diopters into degrees since by definition 1Δ = 1 cm at 1 m. Then the circumference of such a circle would be 360 degrees = 628 cm (or Δ) so 1Δ = .573 degrees.

A prism of 10Δ would deviate light about _____ degrees.

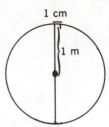

1 cm

1 m

---

796. (1) 3 PD
(2) down

---

797. The segment used in a Kryptok bifocal is 22 mm in diameter. To reduce this diameter the front surface of the bifocal lens may be ground down after fusion. The maximum width of a Kryptok bifocal is (1) _____ and to reduce this width the (2) _____ surface should be ground down.

---

968. weaker

---

969. The average aphakic correction in spectacles is +10.00 D. Spectacle lenses of this power inherently produce aberrations. If a high plus lens is tilted, significant _____ can be induced.
(type of aberration)

109. 90

---

110. The power of a cylinder is 90 degrees from the axis. A lens with the formula $+2.00$ -3.00×90 has $+2.00$ D power at 90 degrees and _____ D power at 180 degrees.

---

281. (1) one
(2) three

---

282. Cycloplegics are potent drugs and should be prescribed with caution. Parents should be instructed to stop medication if side effects, such as rash, fever and erythema develop. Any cycloplegic remaining after the prescribed dosage has been given should be destroyed.

The side effects of cycloplegics may be (1) _____ , (2) _____ , (3) _____ .

---

453. (*Advance to next frame.*)

---

454. Retinoscopy is an objective means of measuring the refractive state of an eye. A light is directed into an eye and the movement of the red reflex thus produced is observed. If the reflex movement (as compared to the movement of the light) is "with," we add plus lenses to neutralize. If the movement of the reflex is "against," we would add _____ lenses to neutralize.

625. 5.73 (or 5)

---

626. The relation of prism diopters to degrees is 1.75Δ = 1 degree or about 2Δ to 1 degree.

If a patient has a 20Δ exophoria, the exophoria is about _____ degrees.

---

797. (1) 22 mm
(2) anterior (or front)

---

798. Kryptok bifocals are low in cost and inconspicuous. Their main disadvantage is the chromatic aberration in adds greater than 2.00 D.

If a patient complained of seeing rings of colors about the print through a +3.00 D add Kryptok bifocal, the _____ of the +3.00 D add explains this complaint.

---

969. astigmatism (or astigmatism of oblique incidence)

---

970. When retinoscoping an aphakic patient, it is important to avoid tipping trial lenses in order to eliminate the induction of _____.

110. −1.00

---

111. If the total power is +8.00 D at 90 degrees and +4.00 D at 180 degrees, we can diagram this lens (+4.00 + 4.00 × 180) as:

_____ D axis (2) _____ degrees or (3) _____ D axis (4) _____ degrees.

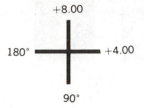

This indicates a cylinder which may be (1)

---

282. (1) fever
(2) rash
(3) erythema (also palpitations, thirst, and dry mucous membranes) } in any order

---

283. The toxicity of cycloplegics is usually caused by large amounts of the solution draining from the eye into the nose via the lacrimal passages. Atropine's toxicity is minimized by prescribing atropine ointment to be used at bedtime daily for three days prior to the refraction.

Toxicity due to atropine ointment should be expected to occur (less/more) frequently than toxicity due to atropine drops.

---

454. minus (or concave)

---

455. A retinoscope consists of a source of illumination and an aperture through a reflecting mirror for observation of the reflex. If the mirror is tilted forward (the same as moving the source of light up) point A will move _____.

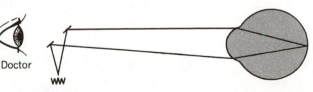

626. 10

---

627. Phorias may be measured by dissociating the eye with a Maddox rod and adding prisms to align the images. A patient fixates on a light while having a Maddox rod in front of OD and sees the images as depicted in Diagram A. Prism base (nasal/temporal) will be necessary to align the images as depicted by Diagram B. (Remember a prism displaces an image toward its apex.)

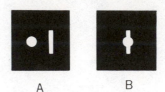

A   B

---

798. chromatic aberration

---

799. The competition among producers of Kryptok bifocals has encouraged low prices and short cuts in techniques of production. As a result there are many Kryptok bifocals which are of low quality with distorted optical qualities.

Kryptok bifocals are of (equal/varying) quality.

---

970. astigmatism (or astigmatism of oblique incidence)

---

971. The high power of aphakic spectacle corrections creates magnification of retinal images. If one eye is aphakic and the other phakic, significant _____ is produced by spectacle correction of the aphakia.

111. (1) −4.00 (3) +4.00 (1 and 2 may
(2) 90 (4) 180 be reversed
with 3 and 4.)

---

112. +5.00 − 5.00 × 45 may be diagrammed: +2.00 − 1.00 × 90 may be diagrammed:

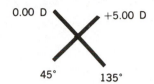

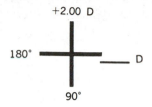

---

283. less

284.

PART IV

MYOPIA, HYPEROPIA, AND ASTIGMATISM

(Advance to next frame.)

---

455. down

---

456. If the retinoscope is tilted to direct the light further down on an eye (having the same effect as moving the light source up), the image (point A) will move down. Point A may or may not be blurred, but its movement will always be in the _____ direction as the movement of the light on the eye of the patient.

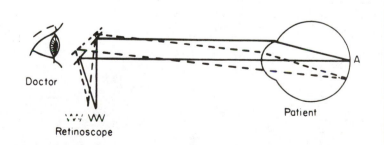

627. temporal

---

628. If a prism base is temporal before an eye, we call the prism direction base out. If the prism base is nasal, we call the prism direction base _____ .

---

799. varying

---

800. The prismatic effect in the illustrated bifocal may be calculated as follows: At the point where the visual axis meets the upper edge of the segment the distance lens provides 1.5Δ base up (5.00 × 0.3). At this point the add provides 2.2Δ base down (2.00 × 1.1). The net prismatic effect through the upper edge of the segment 3 mm below the optical center of the distance correction is (1) _____ prism diopters base (2) _____ .

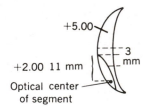

+5.00

+2.00 11 mm

3 mm

Optical center of segment

---

971. aniseikonia

---

972. Image magnification by aphakic spectacles is about 30 percent. Aniseikonia of this amount is most generally (tolerable/intolerable).

112. +1.00

---

113. $+8.50 - 6.50 \times 30$ may be diagrammed:

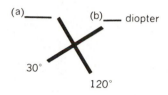

(a)_____   (b)___ diopter

30°

120°

---

284. (*Advance to next frame.*)

---

285. An unaccommodated eye capable of focusing parallel light rays on the retina is termed an emmetropic eye. Such a state is termed emmetropia.

An emmetropic eye uses _____ D accommodation to focus the divergent rays of light from an object 0.5 m away.

---

456. same

---

457. The image on the patient's retina moves in the same direction as the retinoscope light is moved on the patient's eye. This image (the reflex) will appear to the observer to move either in the same direction, with motion, or in an opposite direction, against motion, depending on (1) the refractive state of the patient's eye and (2) the distance the observer is from the patient.

The reflex will be observed to move either the (1) _____ or (2) _____ direction in relation to the image movement on the retina.

628. in

---

629. Esophoria (uncrossed diplopia) is measured with prism base _____.

---

800. (1) 0.7
(2) down

---

801. When prisms are arranged apex to base the image jump, when looking from one to the other, is the same as the image jump produced by a prism equal to their difference. (*Answer space is in the diagram.*)

4^Δ

5^Δ

$= 1^\Delta$
image jump

5^Δ

3^Δ

$= \underline{\hspace{1cm}}^\Delta.$
image jump

---

972. intolerable

---

973. The amount of aniseikonia produced by spectacle correction of monocular aphakia is generally intolerable. Accordingly, monocular aphakic patients who wear spectacle correction of the aphakia require obliteration of the image from the phakic eye. This is accomplished by prescribing a balancing high plus lens for the phakic eye. Spectacle corrected monocular aphakic patients (do/do not) have binocular vision.

113. (a) $+2.00$
(b) $+8.50$

114.

$+3.00$ D

$5°$ ——|—— $+4.00$ D

$95°$

The diagram may be written using a plus cylinder as $+3.00 + 1.00 \times 95$, or using a minus cylinder as $+4.00$ _____ $\times 5$.

---

285. 2.00

---

286. Many factors may cause hypermetropia or myopia, but, as depicted in the diagram, axial differences are one cause.

Axial changes are a major factor in determining the final refractive state. This would imply that the length of a myope's eye is usually _____ than the length of a hyperope's eye.

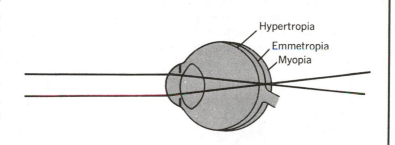

---

457. (1) same (or with)
(2) opposite (or against) } either order

458. As the image A on the retina moves to B we see the reflex focusing at the far point of the patient's eye and moving in a direction _____ both the image on the retina and the direction of the retinoscope's light on the outside of the patient's eye.

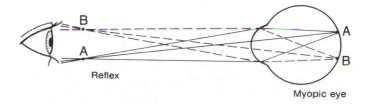

629. out

630. Exophoria (crossed diplopia) is measured with prism base _____ .

---

801. 2

802. When prisms are arranged apex to apex or base to base the image jump, when looking from one to the other, is the same as the image jump produced by a prism equal to the sum of their powers. (*Answer space is in the diagram.*)

4^Δ

5^Δ = 1^Δ image jump

5^Δ

3^Δ = ___$^\Delta$. image jump

---

973. do not

974. High plus spectacle lenses used to correct aphakia produce severe prismatic effects, both horizontal and vertical, when the patient changes his visual axis in respect to the optical center of the lens. In addition, movement of the patient's head produces illusory movement of the environment. Adaptation to aphakic spectacles requires significant efforts to overcome the _____ produced by the lenses.

114. -1.00

115.

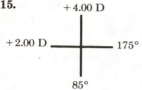

+4.00 D

+2.00 D ——— 175°

85°

The diagram may be written in minus cylinder form as $+4.00 - 2.00 \times 85$, or in plus cylinder form as _____.

---

286. greater (or longer)

287. Parallel light rays are focused on the retina of an emmetropic eye, behind the retina in a hyperopic eye, and in front of the retina in a myopic eye.

Myopia and hypermetropia may be corrected with the appropriate lenses causing parallel rays to focus on the retina.

(1) _____ lenses correct hyperopia (frequently called hypermetropia); (2) _____ lenses correct myopia.

---

458. opposite to

459. If your eye is within the patient's far point you will see "with" motion; if you are outside the far point you will see _____ motion because the light rays have crossed at the far point.

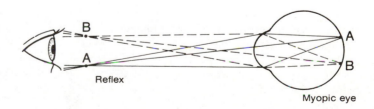

Reflex

Myopic eye

630. in

631. An easy way to remember that exophoria produces crossed diplopia when the images are dissociated is to remember that there is an "X" (or cross) in exophoria, so it is _____ diplopia.

---

802. 5.0

803. When looking through the diagrammed lens an image jump results as the visual axis moves from the area of 1.5Δ base up to the area of 2.5Δ base down total prismatic power. The image jump is the same as suddenly looking through a _____ diopter prism.

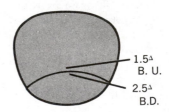

1.5ᐃ
B. U.

2.5ᐃ
B.D.

---

974. prismatic effects

975. A +11.00 D lens is found on refraction to correct an aphakic eye when the trial frame is 15 mm from the eye. The spectacle lens will be 12 mm from the eye. What power spectacle lens will have the same effective power as the +11.00 D found on refraction (to the nearest 1/8 D)?

115. $+2.00 + 2.00 \times 175$

116. It is often necessary, for technical reasons of manufacture, to create a toric surface on the concave side of a meniscus lens. The convex surface of the lens appearing in the drawing measured $+9.00$ D in all meridians, indicating it is a (1) (spherical/toric) surface. On the concave side the 180 degrees meridian measured -5.50 D. The 90 degree meridian is shown in the drawing and measures (2) _____ D, indicating the concave surface to be (3) (spherical/toric).

(sign and power)

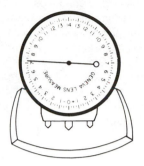

---

287. (1) + (or convex)
(2) − (or concave)

288. Any refractive state other than emmetropia is called ametropia. Myopia and hyperopia are examples of ametropia.

Myopia and hyperopia are conditions of (1) _____.

In myopia parallel rays of light are focused (2) _____ the retina.
In hyperopia parallel rays of light are focused (3) _____ the retina.

---

459. against

460. The observer again sees the reflex at the far point of the patient's eye (which is now behind the eye), so the reflex in this instance will move in the _____ direction as the image on the retina and the retinoscope's light on the outside of the patient's eye.

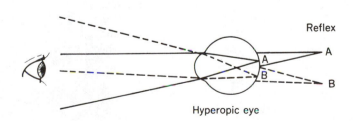

Reflex

A

B

Hyperopic eye

631. crossed

632. Revolving prisms provide an easy method of increasing or decreasing the prisms used to measure phorias. Prisms placed apex to base, if of equal power, provide no prismatic power. If prism A is rotated in relation to prism B, the neutralizing value of *A* is reduced and a measurable prismatic effect is gained. If prism A is changed from the diagram and placed apex to apex with prism B, then the total prismatic power is _____.

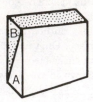

803. 4

804. As the visual axis crosses the segment edge there is image jump unless the optical centers of the distance and add are located at this point. As the visual axis passes the edge of the bifocal segment in A there will be a 6Δ _____.

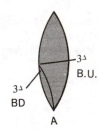

975. +11.37 D

976. A frequent source of difficulty with aphakic corrections is failure to measure vertex distance when refracting. If the vertex distance is specified, any difference between the fit of the spectacles and trial frame can be compensated by a change in the _____ of the lenses.

116. (1) spherical
    (2) −7.25
    (3) toric

117. The surfaces of a lens measure +9.00 D spherical on the front surface, and on the back surface, −7.25 D in the 90 degree meridian, and as shown in the 180 degree meridian. (1) Complete the diagram. (2) Write the formula in minus cylinder form.

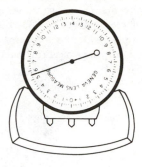

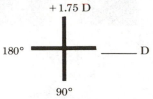

+1.75 D

180°   _____ D

90°

---

288. (1) ametropia
    (2) in front of
    (3) behind

289. Myopia exists when the refractive power of the eye is too great for the length of the eye; thus the rays focus in front of the retina.

    What type of light rays will an uncorrected myopic eye focus on the retina? (parallel/divergent/convergent)

---

460. same

---

461. In retinoscopy at the end point (called neutrality), the pupil of the patient is suddenly filled with light and no motion is observed.

    What motion is observed at neutrality during retinoscopy?

632. power of prism A plus power of prism B

---

633. Quantitation of heterophoria is necessary. The phoria may be conveniently measured with prisms. With the Maddox rod in front of OD the patient sees A. A prism displaces an image toward its apex. A suitable amount of prism base (in/out) OS will change the picture to B.

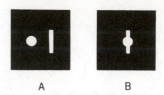

A   B

---

804. image jump

---

805. Image jump occurs when the visual axis crosses the edge of the segment. Any prismatic effect of the lens when the visual axis is stationary and passes through one point in the bifocal is called image displacement. When the visual axis passes as in Figure A there is a net prismatic effect of 2Δ base up producing 2Δ _____ .

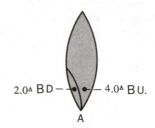

2.0ᐃ BD — 4.0ᐃ BU.

A

---

976. power

---

977. Because of the importance of vertex distance, aphakic spectacles must be constantly kept in precise adjustment. Slight loosening of the frame will result in a change of vision. If aphakic spectacles loosen and the vertex distance of the glasses increases, the effective power of the lenses will be (increased/decreased).

117. (1) +3.50

(2) +3.50 − 1.75 ×180

---

118. One lens measures +1.50 + 2.00 × 90, and another lens measures +3.50 − 2.00 × 180. These two lenses have identical refractive power expressed in a different manner, since they are ground in a different manner. The sign of the cylinder in the first lens is plus and in the second minus, but the cylinders are _____ in power.

---

289. divergent

---

290. A myopic eye has a fixed far point which is determined by the amount of myopia. The far point is that point which the unaccommodated eye can focus on the retina; hence its distance from the eye is the reciprocal of the refractive error of the eye. The far point of this unaccommodated myopic eye is _____ m(s).

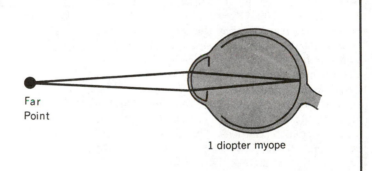

1 diopter myope

---

461. No motion

---

462. If the observer were at infinity (or at least 20 feet), a myopic eye would always show an against motion of the reflex and a hyperopic eye would show a with motion of the reflex. Since the observer usually works at either 66 cm or 50 cm, one of these distances becomes the point at which neutrality is sought. If an eye showed neutrality of the reflex at 50 cm, this would be the far point and the patient would be known to be a (1) _____ D (2) (myope/emmetrope/hyperope).

633. out

---

634. You will remember that if a prism is placed so that its base is temporally, we refer to this as prism base out; if nasally, prism base (1) _____.

Prism base out measures esophoria. Prism (2) _____ measures exophoria.

---

805. image displacement

---

806. Image displacement may be calculated as follows: In a +3.00 D lens, a +2.00 D Kryptok segment is placed so that the top edge of this 22 mm segment (with its optical center 11 mm down) is 3 mm below the center of the lens. To find the net prismatic power 6 mm below the top edge of the bifocal, consider the point 9 mm below the optical center of the distance correction. There are $(0.9 \times +3.00)$ 2.7Δ B.U. resulting from the distance portion of the lens. The segment results in (11 minus 6 mm) or $0.5 \times +2.00 = 1.0Δ$ B.D. at the stated point. Net prism power is (1) _____ Δ base (2) _____ 6 mm below the top edge of the segment.

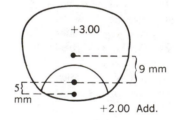

---

977. increased

---

978. As has been shown, the high power of aphakic spectacles produces significant problems for the patient. Some of these problems can be minimized by the use of aspheric lenses, or lenses ground selectively to alter the marked difference between the center of the lens and the periphery. It is not practical to manufacture iseikonic lenses for aphakic patients, so all aphakic spectacle lenses produce _____ of the retinal image.

118. the same (or equal)

---

119. Mathematically changing a lens formula from one expressing the cylinder as a plus cylinder to one expressing the cylinder as minus (or vice versa) is called **transposition.** If the formula of a lens with a plus cylinder is changed to a formula incorporating a minus cylinder, the formula has been

_____.

---

290. 1

---

291. An uncorrected 4.00 D myope has a far point of (1) _____ cm. When he accommodates 2.00 D this far point moves in to (2) _____ cm.

---

462. (1) 2.00
    (2) myope

---

463. Neutrality of the reflex occurs when the far point of the patient's eye coincides with the cornea of your eye. When the far point is 1 mm from your cornea, you require 1000.00 D accommodation to see any detail of the reflex, so, instead of seeing "against" motion you see only a red reflex or nothing. This red color without motion is called

_____.

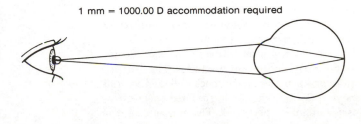

1 mm = 1000.00 D accommodation required

634. (1) in
(2) base in

---

635. Revolving prisms are commercially available and appear as indicated. The figures and line indicate the prism diopters and base of the prism. These auxilliary lenses are conveniently accessible on a phoropter as well. In the photo the patient reports the targets aligned and thus has (1) _____ Δ (2) _____ phoria.

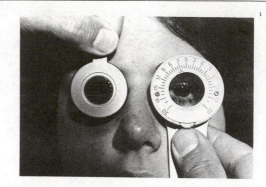

---

806. (1) 1.7
(2) up

---

807. If the lenses prescribed are approximately equal OU, the vertical prismatic power resulting from the bifocal is unimportant, for it will be (equal/unequal) OU when looking down.

---

978. magnification

---

979. Correction of aphakia by spectacles creates problems for the refractionist and optician as well as for the patient. Particular attention must be paid to astigmatism of oblique incidence and vertex distance. Astigmatism of oblique incidence can be controlled by careful attention to the pantoscopic tilt of both trial frame and spectacles. The distance in millimeters between the back cell of the trial frame and the eye should be specified on prescriptions for aphakic spectacles. This measurement is known as the _____.

119. transposed

---

120. A formula is transposed by: (1) algebraically adding the power of the sphere and cylinder and using the result as the new sphere; (2) reversing the sign of the cylinder, keeping the power the same, and (3) changing the axis 90 degrees. Transpose $+4.00 + 2.00 \times 90$.

---

291. (1) 25
(2) 16.66

---

292. An uncorrected myope of 5.00 D who has 2.00 D of accommodation can see objects clearly from (1) _____ cm to (2) _____ cm from his eye.

---

463. neutrality

---

464. A retinoscopist (with no lenses on patient) working at 66.66 cm will observe an against motion when retinoscoping a 2.00 D myopic eye. When retinoscoping the same eye at a working distance of 50 cm he observes neutrality. When the retinoscopist moves to 40 cm he will observe a(n) _____ reflex motion from this eye.

635. (1) 3
(2) exo

---

636. With the Maddox rod over one eye and the revolving prism in front of the other, prismatic power is increased in the proper direction until the patient reports the light to be on the line. If the patient sees A (with Maddox rod over right eye), the patient has (1) _____ phoria and prism base (2) _____ must be used for measurement.

A

---

807. equal

---

808. If there is anisometropia (unequal refractive states in the two eyes), a vertical prismatic effect may become a problem on downward gaze. The illustration demonstrates the vertical prismatic effect occurring when a patient having 1.00 D myopia OD and 1.00 D hyperopia OS reads through a point 8 mm below the optical center in each lens. The net prismatic effect of the two lenses at this point is the sum of the two if different in base directions or the difference if base direction is the same. The net diagrammed is _____ Δ base down OD or base up OS.

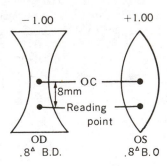

---

979. vertex distance

---

980. Errors in vertex distance can be minimized by the technique of over-refraction. A pair of spectacles approximating the patients fit and having high plus spheres (about +12.00 D) is placed on the patient, and, in a lens carrier attached to the frame, the astigmatic correction found by retinoscopy and cross cylinder verification is added anterior to the high plus spectacle lens. Spherical lenses are then added to the combination until best distant visual acuity is achieved. The prescription written is the sum of all the lenses before the eye with the vertex distance specified. The technique of (1) _____ in aphakia requires the use of spectacles containing (2) _____ .

120. $+6.00 - 2.00 \times 180$

---

121. Transpose $+5.00 - 1.00 \times 45$.

---

292. (1) 20 } either
(2) 14.28 } order

---

293. One goal of refraction is to place the far point of an unaccommodated eye at infinity, thus focusing parallel rays of light on the retina. Plus lenses (the same effect on the far point as accommodation) bring the far point closer to the eye while _____ lenses push the far point away from the eye.

---

464. with

---

465. An astigmatic error can be seen much better using a line rather than a circular source of light, so any meridian can be neutralized separately. A convenient instrument of this type is the streak retinoscope. A retinoscope having a line image which can be rotated to any meridian is called a _____.

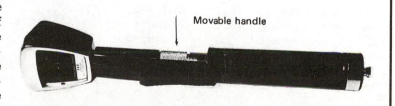

Movable handle

636. (1) exo
     (2) in

---

637. If the patient sees A (with Maddox rod OD), he has (1) _____ phoria which can be measured by adding prism base (2) _____.

A

---

808. 1.6

---

809. If there is anisometropia and bifocals are worn, the vertical imbalance on downward gaze may be solved in two ways—either the position of the optical center of the segment may be altered or prism power may be added to the segment. The bifocal segment of the lens before the more myopic eye of an anisometrope should provide more prism base (up/down) than the segment of the other lens to compensate for the prismatic difference in the reading position.

---

980. (1) over refraction
     (2) high plus spheres

---

981. Refraction of aphakic patients is most accurately accomplished by astigmatic verification of retinoscopy by cross cylinder and spherical verification by over-refracting. The use of astigmatic dials for refracting aphakic patients (is/is not) recommended.

121. $+4.00 + 1.00 \times 135$

---

122. The formula of a bifocal is written, for example, $+2.00 - 2.00 \times 135$ with $+1.50$ add. This indicates that there is _____ D more plus power in the bifocal segment than in the distance portion of this lens.

---

293. minus

---

294. If the far point is 0.5 m a -2.00 D lens will push this far point back to 20 feet (20 feet is regarded as infinity).

If the far point is 0.33 m the lens required is _____ to push this far point to 20

(sign and power)
feet.

---

465. streak retinoscope

---

466. All of the explanations to this point have concerned rays which are divergent from the retinoscope. If the light is convergent when it strikes the eye, all relative movements are reversed. The possibility of changing the vergence of rays is included in the streak retinoscope. The handle which turns the streak has an up and down position. The up position is usually used and produces divergent rays. If you prefer the opposite image (some doctors prefer to use "with" motion at all times), you simply lower the handle and reverse the vergence of rays. The end point is still neutrality.

If the handle is in an up position, the emergent rays are _____.

637. (1) eso
(2) out

638. Vertical phorias are denoted by the eye which is higher in the dissociated state. The eye which is higher is termed hyperphoric. If the right eye is higher, the patient has a right hyperphoria. If the right eye is lower, the patient has a _____ .

809. up

810. The Univis bifocals were the first to offer variable positions of optical centers in the segment. This is accomplished by cutting the segment in different portions and filling in the remainder of the countersink with crown glass. The net prismatic effect through the reading part of lenses A and B is (the same/different) at any corresponding point.

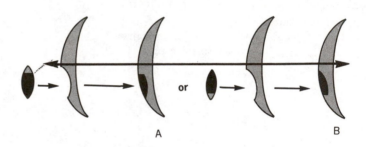

A   or   B

981. is not

982. If a plus lens is moved closer to the eye, its effective power (increases/decreases).

122. 1.50

123. The amount of add of a fused bifocal segment (can/cannot) be determined with the lens gauge.

---

294. −3.00 D

295. The chief complaint of an uncorrected myope who has a far point of 0.5 m will be _____ .

---

466. divergent

467. The retinoscopist may select any distance at which to work, but, in general, 66 cm or 50 cm is conventional. Use the shorter distance if your arms are short to facilitate handling lenses. If using 50 cm, neutral retinoscopy without lenses means the eye is 2.00 D myopic and an emmetropic eye requires +2.00 D for neutrality. Therefore the total power must be adjusted by −2.00 D if using 50 cm.

If you select 66 cm, you will then adjust the total power you find at the neutralization point by

_____ .
(sign and diopters)

638. left hyperphoria

639. When one eye deviates upward while the other eye remains aligned on a target the image of the target will fall on the upper portion of the retina of the deviating eye and remain on the fovea of the fixating eye. What portion of the retina of the upward deviating eye will be stimulated while the other eye fixates a target? (Upper/Lower)

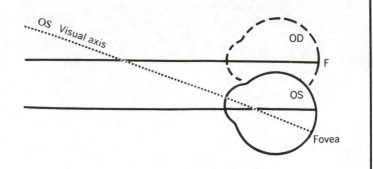

810. different

811. The Univis bifocal technique has just been described. If technique A results in the type bifocal B, what type bifocal does technique C produce? (*Sketch your answer.*)

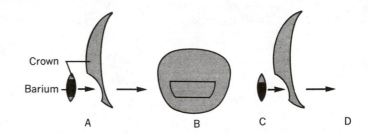

982. decreases

983. A contact lens used to correct a given aphakic eye will have (more plus/less plus) than the spectacle lens required to correct the eye.

123. cannot

---

124. The base curve of a bifocal is the curve ground on the segment side of the lens, whether or not the other surface is toric. In a fused bifocal, the anterior surface is the _____ .

---

295. blurring of objects at any distance greater than 0.5 m from him (this or equivalent)

---

296. A 4.00 D myope who has 2.00 D accommodation will be able to see objects clearly that are (1) _____ cm to (2) _____ cm from the eye.

---

467. − 1.50

---

468. Accurate retinoscopy depends on light passing along the visual axis. If the patient had a cycloplegic drug, occlude one eye and have the patient look directly at your retinoscope light. If the patient has not been cyclopleged, place some additional plus before the fixing eye and have the patient view a fixation light at 20 feet. Then align the retinoscope with his visual axis as closely as possible, using your OD to retinoscope his OD and your OS for his OS. In a noncyclopleged patient you would examine his OD using your (1) _____ and his OS using your (2) _____ .

639. Upper

---

640. Since a fixation image strikes a point above the fovea of an upward deviating eye, the patient will report this image as being (higher/lower) than the image seen by the fixating eye.

811.

---

812. The net prismatic power of the reading portion of the bifocal may be altered by incorporating prism into the bifocal add or by varying the position of the _____ of the segment.

---

983. more plus

---

984. An aphakic eye is corrected by a spectacle lens of +10.00 D, 12 mm vertex distance. The power of a correcting contact lens will be approximately _____ D. $(\Delta D = sD^2)$

124. base curve

---

125. In a fused bifocal the _____ surface is the base curve.

---

296. (1) 25 } either
(2) 16 2/3 } order

---

297. The far point (*punctum remotum* or pr) of a myope is determined by his myopia and the near point (*punctum proximum* or pp) is determined by the amount of myopia plus the amount of accommodation. If the myopia is high, his range of clear vision will be small.

An uncorrected 10.00 D myope who has 10.00 D of accommodation sees clearly from his pr of (1) _____ to his pp of (2) _____ .

---

468. (1) OD
(2) OS

---

469. The diagram shows the appearance of the streak and reflex in "with" motion. If the working distance (with handle up) is 66 cm and you note this reflex, you could say this patient is (disregarding astigmatism) less than (1) _____ D myopic, but could be (2) _____ or (3) _____ .

(All frames refer to divergent rays produced by the up position of the retinoscope handle.)

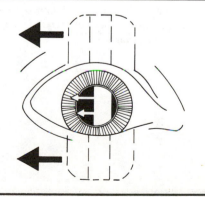

249

640. lower

---

641. The Maddox rod is turned to the vertical position so a horizontal line will be seen and the vertical phoria is measured with revolving prisms. If the Maddox rod is in front of OD and the patient sees A, the image strikes the lower part of the right retina and it is projected above the left image. He has a _____ hyperphoria.

A

---

812. optical center

---

813. One type of bifocal suitable for incorporating any direction prismatic power in the segment is the Panoptik (Bausch & Lomb). The prism pictured here is base (1) _____, but a prism with its base in (2) _____ direction may be attained with the Panoptik bifocal.

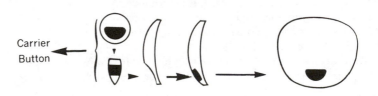

Carrier Button

---

984. +11.25

---

985. According to Knapp's rule, spectacle correction of aphakia (does/does not) produce magnification of the retinal image.

125. anterior

---

126. The lens in the drawing measures the same in all meridians. The anterior surface of this lens is (1) (spherical/toric) and measures (2) _____ .
  (sign and power)

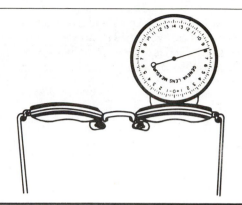

---

297. (1) 10 cm
  (2) 5 cm

---

298. If the pr of a myope is 12.5 cm and he has 12.00 D of accommodation, uncorrected he will see objects clearly at (1) _____ cm when not accommodating and is (2) _____ D myopic. His pp, uncorrected, is (3) _____ cm.

---

469. (1) 1.5
  (2) hyperopic ⎫ either
  (3) emmetropic ⎰ order

---

470. "Against" motion is diagrammed. If your working distance is 66 cm (and the sleeve of the retinoscope is in the up position), this patient will be (1) _____ and requires a lens greater than (2) _____ .

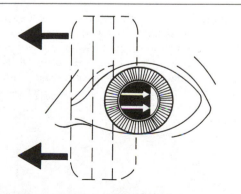

641. left

---

642. A patient reports the Maddox rod image seen by a hyperphoric eye to be (1) (higher/lower) than the image of the fixating eye. The hyperphoric eye requires prism base (2) _____ to align the images.

---

813. (1) up
(2) any

---

814. Another method of incorporating prismatic power in the bifocal is the slab-off technique. This method produces prism base up in the reading area.

First a dummy lens is cemented to the anterior surface of the bifocal.

The cross-hatched area represents a _____.

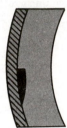

---

985. does

---

986. Magnification of the retinal image in spectacle corrected aphakia is about 30 percent. The closer the lens to the eye, the less magnification of the retinal image. An aphakic eye corrected by a contact lens has about a +7 percent magnification of the retinal image. In aphakia, contact lenses provide a more normal sized _____ than spectacles.

126. (1) spherical
(2) +8.25

---

127. The drawing depicts a lens being measured in the 180 degree meridian. This is the same lens shown in the previous frame where the anterior surface measured +8.25 D. The back surface power of the 180 degree meridian as shown is (1) _____ D, and the lens power in the
(sign and power)
180 degree meridian is (2) _____ D.
(sign and power)

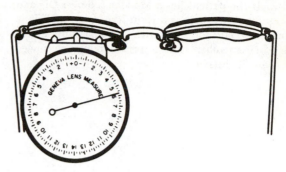

---

298. (1) 12.5
(2) 8.00
(3) 5

---

299. At birth myopia is a rare condition; hyperopia is the usual condition (2.00 to 3.00 D). During growth hyperopia decreases (or myopia increases). The average child of age eight is only mildly hyperopic (about 1.00 D).

A child myopic at age three would be expected to be _____ when adult.
(refractive state)

---

470. (1) myopic
(2) −1.50 D

---

471. The reflex will vary in brightness, size and speed as lenses are added. In a given case, the reflex will be brighter, move faster, and be smaller as neutrality is approached. These characteristics are of interest only in estimating how large a step to use in changing lenses. The rule is:

A brighter, faster, smaller reflex than observed with the prior lens means neutrality is (closer/ farther away).

642. (1) lower
(2) down

643. If the patient has a Maddox rod over OD and sees Figure A, he has a right hyperphoria. This is measured and corrected with prism base (up, down) OD. (Remember that a prism moves an image toward its apex.)

A

814. dummy lens

815. Part of the dummy and lens is then ground away (slabbed-off) (A), then the posterior lens is ground away (B), and finally the dummy is removed leaving (C) with base up prism over only _____.

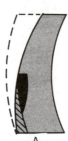 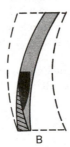 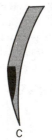

A   B   C

986. retinal image

987. Patients with monocular aphakia and good vision in the unoperated eye usually find it impossible to wear a spectacle uniocular aphakic correction because of the optical aniseikonia. The size difference present when a contact lens is worn to correct the aphakia is usually tolerated. An excellent indication for the use of a contact lens is _____.

127. (1) −5.75
(2) +2.50

128. The drawing shows the lens just seen in the previous frame. This measurement is at the 90 degree meridian. The reading is

(1) _____ D for this
<u>(sign and power)</u>

posterior surface. The surface power at 180 degrees was −5.75 D. This is a (2) <u>(toric/spherical)</u> surface.

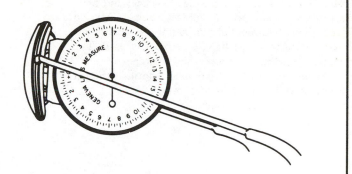

299. myopic

300. The refractive system of the eye has many variants, including corneal and lenticular refraction, depth of the anterior chamber, and axial length of the eye. All of these variants make genetics of refraction a difficult problem. Mild myopia is usually considered to be a dominant trait. If both parents have mild myopia, you would expect <u>(more than half/less than half)</u> of their children to be myopic.

471. closer

472. When the refractive error is neutralized by lenses at a given working distance the pupil is suddenly filled with light. The refractionist can easily check this neutral point by moving forward a few inches, then back a few inches. As he moves forward within the far point of the patient's eye (with handle up) he would expect a(n) (1) _____ motion; as he then backs away, increasing his working distance, he would expect a(n) (2) _____ motion.

643. down

---

644. Heterophorias (or phorias), vertical and horizontal, are measured at 20 feet using a fixation light. The fixation light is simply a small light bulb. At near, a pen light is frequently used. The Maddox rod can be used in both instances.

To measure distant and near phorias (using a Maddox rod and revolving prisms) a _____ is a suitable fixation point.

---

815. the reading area

---

816. Be very cautious about prescribing prisms for anyone. Give the prisms only when absolutely necessary, and, even then, have the patient try some temporary clip-on prisms before the final prescription is written. If prisms seem absolutely necessary you should _____ .

---

987. monocular aphakia

---

988. Aberrations of lenses increase with the increase in lens power. Patients wearing aphakic spectacles have clear vision only through the center of the lenses plus a lens induced ring scotoma as well as image magnification. All these optical problems are practically eliminated by contact lenses and intraocular lenses. Contact lens correction is much superior to spectacle correction of _____ .

128. (1) −6.75
 (2) toric

129. The anterior lens surface measures +8.25 D in all meridians. The posterior surface measures −5.25 D in the 180 degree meridian and −6.25 D in the 90 degree meridian. The formula of this lens is _____ .

300. more than half

301. A given trait, such as myopia, is determined by the genes of the parent. Myopia below 6.00 D is usually dominant; above 6.00 D (high myopia) recessive, requiring that both genes be affected.

Mo	*Mm*	*mm*	*mo*	*M* = dominant for low myopia
low	low	high	no	*m* = recessive for high myopia
myope	myope	myope	myopia	*o* = no myopia

If both parents had high myopia (all/none) of the offspring would be expected to be myopic.

472. (1) with
 (2) against

473. Just as in neutralization of lenses where apparent with motion was neutralized by plus lenses and apparent against motion was neutralized with minus lenses, so in retinoscopy with motion is always neutralized with _____ lenses and against motion is always neutralized with _____ lenses.

644. light (fixation light or equivalent)

645. The usual heterophoria measures 0 to 2Δ exophoria when the patient is fixating at 20 feet. When the patient fixates at near (33.33 cm) the average is 3 to 6Δ exophoria. Although these are the averages, many values well outside these measurements may be considered physiologic for an asymptomatic patient. If a patient were 1Δ exophoric at distance and 7Δ exophoric at near and asymptomatic, would the horizontal phorias be abnormal?

816. let the patient try a temporary clip-on pair

817. The type of bifocal prescribed should be consistent with the patient's needs. If near work predominates, a large field at near is needed. The Executive (American Optical) bifocal is a one-piece bifocal providing such a field. The Executive bifocal is suitable when work is mainly at (1) _____ but not when work is mainly at (2) _____.

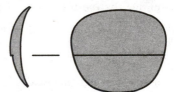

988. aphakia

989. A lens placed within the eye of an aphakic patient will have (1) (more/less) power than a contact lens used to correct the same eye's aphakia, and will produce (2) (more/less) magnification of the retinal image than the contact lens.

129. $+3.00 - 1.00 \times 180$ (or $+2.00 + 1.00 \times 90$)

---

130. If a lens with the following surface measurements were a fused bifocal, what would be the base curve?

Anterior surface $= +8.25$ D

Posterior surface $= \begin{array}{l} -5.25 \text{ D in horizontal meridian} \\ -6.25 \text{ D in vertical meridian} \end{array}$

---

301. all

---

302. Two types of myopia exist. A mildly myopic eye is an essentially healthy eye with a refractive error usually under 6.00 D. Pathologic myopia has many associated physical changes, ranging from a small myopic crescent above the disc to a detached retina, with intervening changes such as liquefied vitreous, extensive choroidal changes often involving the macula, and posterior staphylomas.

A myope greater than _____ D could be expected to have or develop some or all of the above changes.

---

473. (1) plus
(2) minus

---

474. The illustration shows (1) _____ motion and indicates (2) _____ lenses must be added to give neutrality. (Handle of retinoscope is in the usual up position.)

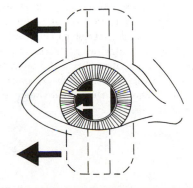

645. no

---

646. X is the usual abbreviation for exophoria at distance and X′ for exophoria at near. The following prisms measured the horizontal phorias:

> 6Δ base in at distance
> 2Δ base in at near

The phorias would be recorded as (1) _____,
(2) _____.

---

817. (1) near
    (2) distance

---

818. Special needs can frequently be met with special bifocals. Carpenters, whose work frequently requires looking up for close work, may require a bifocal add in the upper part of the lens.

    This lens would provide clear vision in what near fields?

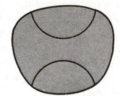

---

989. (1) more
    (2) less

---

990. Intraocular lens implantation is an additional technique used for the correction of aphakia. The lens may be positioned anterior to the iris (in the plane of the iris), or posterior to the iris (in the site of the removed crystalline lens). An intraocular lens placed in front of the iris will need (more/less) power to correct the eye than an intraocular lens placed behind the iris.

130. +8.25 D

---

131. The drawing shows the upper portion of a one piece bifocal being measured. This measures (1) _____ D and will be a different mea-
(sign and power)
surement from the lower anterior segment measurement. The base curve of this lens is (2) _____ D.
(sign and power)

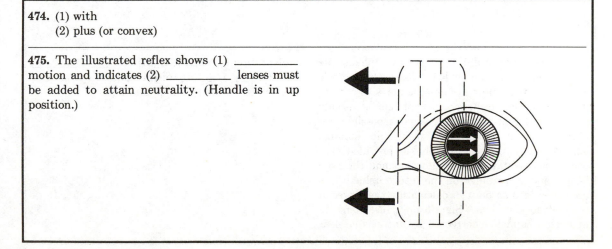

---

302. 6.00

---

303. Myopia under 6.00 D is usually inherited as a (1) _____ trait, while high myopia is usually a (2) _____ trait.

---

474. (1) with
(2) plus (or convex)

---

475. The illustrated reflex shows (1) _____ motion and indicates (2) _____ lenses must be added to attain neutrality. (Handle is in up position.)

646. (1) 6Δ X $\Big\}$ either
(2) 2Δ X′ $\Big\}$ order

---

647. Esophoria is frequently abbreviated E for distance and E′ for near.

6Δ base out for distance = (1) _____ $\Big\}$ (Phoria is
3Δ base out for near = (2) _____ $\Big\}$ recorded).

---

818. Upper and lower

---

819. Adds greater in power than +2.00 D and adds of large diameter produce chromatic aberration if of the fused type. The one-piece bifocal, such as the _____ with the large segment, minimizes this chromatic aberration.

---

990. less

---

991. Aniseikonia prohibits monocular aphakic patients from having binocular vision with spectacle correction. The amount of aniseikonia with contact lens correction of monocular aphakia is usually tolerable so that binocular vision is possible. Intraocular lens implantation results in minimal aniseikonia in monocular aphakia provided that the refractive state of the fellow eye and the axial length and K readings of the future aphakic eye are taken into account in calculating the power of the intraocular lens. Significant aniseikonia in monocular aphakia corrected by intraocular lens implantation is possible if the (1) _____ and (2) _____ of the aphakic eye are not determined before lens implantation.

131. (1) +6.50
(2) +6.50

---

132. The drawing shows the measurement of the segment area of a one piece bifocal. The upper surface measurement was +6.50 D. The difference represents the add of the bifocal. The bifocal add is _____ D.

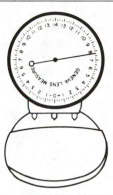

---

303. (1) dominant
(2) recessive

---

304. A rapid increase in myopia has prognostic implications. There is no proven therapy for this progressive myopia, frequently termed malignant myopia.

A child found to require an additional −1.00 D every six months for two years or more would be considered to have _____.

---

475. (1) against
(2) minus

---

476. The streak retinoscope is particularly adaptable for the measurement of astigmatism. The knurled handle allows rotation of the streak so that any meridian may be examined.

What meridians can be measured with the streak retinoscope utilizing the movable handle?

647. (1) 6ΔE
(2) 3ΔE′

648. Vertical prisms, 6Δ or more, before an eye will dissociate the images so that the horizontal phoria may be measured with accommodation fixed. For example, to measure a horizontal phoria while controlling accommodation, a dissociating prism (6Δ) base down OD produces the images as in Diagram 1. (E is the fixation target.) (The upper E is seen by the right eye because of the 6Δ B.D. OD.) Prism base _____ is needed to align the E's as in Diagram 2.

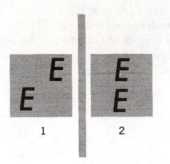

819. Executive

820. Despite the theoretical advantages of certain types of bifocals, a good rule is "to leave well enough alone." If a patient has been happy with the bifocal he is wearing, prescribe the same type when a change in correction is necessary.

If a patient had previously been comfortable wearing a +2.00 D Kryptok bifocal and needs a +2.50 D add, you would probably recommend what type bifocal?

991. (1) axial length ⎫ either
(2) K readings ⎭ order

992. Ultrasonography is used to determine axial length. This measurement and K readings plus knowledge of the type of intraocular lens to be used and the refractive state of the fellow eye are necessary to calculate the (1) _____ of the intraocular lens implanted in monocular aphakia in order to minimize (2) _____.

132. 1.25

---

133. The added power of the segment in a one piece bifocal is determined by the difference in _____ of the two areas of the surface.

---

304. progressive (or malignant) myopia

---

305. The correction of myopia (without astigmatism) is simple. Simply add minus lenses until the best visual acuity at 20 feet is attained. No further minus lenses should be given, for the additional minus would only stimulate accommodation and not improve visual acuity.

   The goal of refraction of a myope is to move the far point of the eye to (1) _____ by the use of (2) _____ lenses.

---

476. All

---

477. When the streak is on axis the streak and line will form _____ line just as was the case with hand neutralization of cylinders.

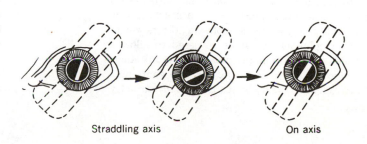

Straddling axis   On axis

648. out

649. Dissociation may be produced simply by prisms placed with base perpendicular to the direction in which heterophoria will be measured. For example, to measure a horizontal phoria, 6Δ base down in front of the right eye might produce Figure A with the upper E being the image seen in the right eye. Additional prism base _____ would be needed to align the E's so that one is directly above the other and thus measure the horizontal phoria.

820. Kryptok

821. Consider a patient whose amplitude of accommodation is 1.00 D. Using maximal accommodation the patient sees clearly through his distance correction from infinity (his far point) to 100 cm. Through a +2.00 D add he can see clearly from 50 cm, without accommodating to 33.33 cm when accommodating maximally. This leaves an intermediate zone, even when utilizing maximum accommodation for distance, from (1) _____ to (2) _____ in which clear vision is not possible using either the distance or near portions of the lenses.

992. (1) power
(2) aniseikonia

993. Intraocular lenses are spherical. Astigmatism may be preexisting or produced by cataract surgery. Additionally, in monocular aphakia, the power of the intraocular lens must be adjusted to allow a spectacle correction approximating the spectacle correction of the fellow eye. An eye containing an intraocular lens is thus seldom exactly _____.

266

133. curvature (or surface measurement)

134. The drawing shows the vertical measurement of a one piece bifocal. The anterior surface measured $+6.50$ D in upper and $+7.75$ D in segment. The horizontal measurement is -6.50 D. Write the formula for this lens including the add.

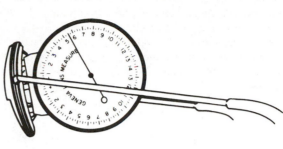

305. (1) 20 feet (considered infinity)
(2) concave (or minus)

306. When a myope removes his glasses he retreats into a world of formless blurs, seeing clearly only those objects which are within his far point. It is no small change when glasses are placed on a child whose previous world extended, only, say 25 cm from him. Similarly, once the myope sees well he is severely handicapped if glasses are lost or broken. You may wish to teach your myopic patients to form a pinhole with their forefinger to see in such emergencies. The familiar sight of a myope squeezing his lids together to find his glasses is a useful maneuver, for he is creating a _____ effect with closure of his lids.

477. one continuous (straight or parallel)

478. Straddling to determine the axis is usually easier when utilizing with motion. With motion, if not present, can be obtained by dropping the handle down to produce convergent rays (thus changing against motion to with motion).

Rotate the streak until the axis is identified and note the greater with or against motion in one axis, then carefully identify the axis by rotating the streak back and forth until the reflex and streak are aligned. Back and forth rotation of the streak, which is done to find the exact axis, is called _____.

649. out

---

650. The vertical phorias are not conveniently measured utilizing horizontally dissociating prisms because a large amount of prismatic power is frequently necessary to dissociate horizontally.

Measurement of the vertical phorias is better accomplished utilizing the _____ for dissociation rather than horizontally dissociating prisms.

---

821. (1) 50 cm ⎫ either
⠀⠀⠀⠀(2) 100 cm ⎭ order

---

822. The intermediate distances in which vision is not clear through either a distance or near correction can be cleared with trifocals (lenses with an add for near and a separate add for intermediate distance). The intermediate add is usually one-half the power of the near add. If the near add is $+2.25$ D, the intermediate add will usually be _____.

---

993. emmetropic

994.

PART XIV

BRIEF REVIEW

(*Advance to next frame.*)

134. $+1.00 \;\; -1.00 \times 90$ (or plano $+1.00 \times 180$)
with $+1.25$ add

---

135. A one piece bifocal has the following measurements:

- $+6.25$ D upper
- $+7.50$ D in add portion
- -6.25 D in 180 degree meridian
- -5.25 D in 90 degree meridian

The base curve of this bifocal is _____ D.
$\underset{\text{(sign and power)}}{}$

---

306. pinhole

---

307. Atropine instilled in one eye will prevent binocular near vision, which is claimed by some to be the cause of progressive myopia. The evidence for this is poor and the use of atropine to prevent binocular near vision is not recommended.

The above theory contends that _____ close work causes progressive myopia.

---

478. straddling

---

479. Net retinoscopy refers to the findings after adjustment for the working distance. Gross retinoscopy is the finding without adjustment for the working distance.

If the working distance is 50 cm, the net retinoscopy will be _____ D less hyperopic or more myopic than the gross retinoscopy.

650. Maddox rod

---

651. Most patients have a measurable tendency to keep the eyes aligned on one object before they yield to diplopia. This fusional reserve can be measured utilizing the revolving prism.

The amount of prismatic power which can be overcome while still maintaining binocular vision is a measure of _____.

---

822. 1.12 D

---

823. Which of the lenses diagrammed below provides the wider field of clear intermediate vision (1) _____ and which the wider field of clear near vision (2) _____?

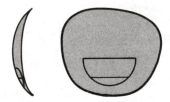
Straight-type fused trifocal

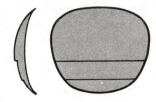
Executive trifocal

---

994. (*Advance to next frame.*)

---

995. A 46-year-old male complains of blurred near vision. His present single vision distance glasses are:

$$\begin{array}{ll} OD + 1.00 - 2.00 \times 45 \\ OS + 2.00 - 2.00 \times 135 \end{array} \quad V_{cc} \quad \begin{array}{l} OD\ 20/20 \\ OS\ 20/20 \end{array}$$

A +0.25 over the present prescription blurs the 20/20 line with either eye. The probable diagnosis is _____.

135. +6.25

---

136. We often want to find the power of a lens. Earlier you saw how this could be done by neutralization when you placed a +2.00 sphere over a −2.00 sphere and observed that with this combination there was no _____ .

---

307. binocular

---

308. Bifocals have been recommended by some as treatment for progressive myopia, but no convincing statistics are available which substantiate that the use of bifocals arrests progressive myopia. Bifocals have little to recommend them, since the uncorrected myope normally requires (more/less) accommodation than the emmetrope at any near distance.

---

479. 2.00

---

480. When gross retinoscopy shows +3.00 − 4.00 × 90 at working distance of 50 cm, the net retinoscopy will be +1.00 − 4.00 × 90. This indicates the cylindrical portion of the correction (is/is not) changed by the working distance adjustment.

651. fusional reserve

652. To measure one aspect of fusional reserve, have the patient fixate on a 20/40 letter at 20 feet and increase prism base in (using revolving prisms) until the patient reports diplopia. Prism base in is then reduced until single vision is reported. The prismatic powers which result in these two end points are recorded as the break point and recovery point of divergence fusional reserve (or amplitude of divergence) at distance. Divergence fusional reserve is measured with prism base _____ .

823. (1) Executive
     (2) Executive

824. Trifocal lenses provide three relatively fixed focal distances. An ideal lens for a presbyope should provide him with clear vision at any focal distance up to his near point. Spectacle lenses are now available which gradually increase in power from distance to full near add. Such lenses do not have demarcation lines between different powers. The higher the near add, the closer the focal distance of the middle segment of a trifocal. Spectacles with a gradual increase of power from distance to full near add are more useful for patients who require ($+2.50/+1.25$) add for reading.

995. presbyopia

996. Placement of plus lenses in front of an emmetropic patient creates an artificial myopia. The patient will not be able to see clearly past this new closer far point. If $+2.00$ D lenses are placed before an emmetrope he cannot see clearly past _____ inches.

136. apparent motion

---

137. A minus cylinder such as -3.00×90 can be written as plano -3.00×90 (plano means 0 net curvature).
   Fill in diopters.

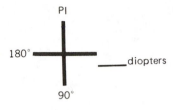

PI

180°   _____ diopters

90°

---

308. less

---

309. Pseudomyopia or accommodative spasm must be differentiated from true myopia. Close observation of the pupil size while the patient is attempting to read the distant chart may give you a clue, for if there is accommodative spasm, causing pseudomyopia, the pupil may become smaller as more accommodation is used. A pupil which changes size while fixation and illumination are unchanged makes _____ a real possibility.

---

480. is not

---

481. When the handle of the streak retinoscope is in the usual up position (1) _____ rays are produced; in the down position (2) _____ rays are produced.

652. in

---

653. Base in prism is increased until the break point is reached and the patient sees double (16Δ), then reduced until he sees singly (8Δ). This is recorded as divergence fusional reserve 16Δ/8Δ.

Divergence fusional reserve 24Δ/16Δ means 24Δ base (1) _____ caused (2) _____, and at 16Δ base (3) _____ he regained (4) _____ .

---

824. +2.50

---

825. Patients who require a relatively low add for reading generally have enough remaining accommodation that trifocals are not necessary. Will the same patients benefit from a variable addition type lens?

---

996. 20

---

997. A +1.00 D sphere over the distance lenses allows the patient to read the 14/14 line without difficulty (at 14 inches). Through the above lens combination he can read the 14/14 line as it is pushed toward him until it reaches 8 inches. The farthest point he can see the print will be _____ inches.

137. -3.00 D

138.

This diagram written in plus cylinder form would be $-3.00 + (1)$ _____ $\times$ (2) _____ .

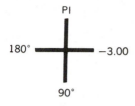

---

309. pseudomyopia (or accommodative spasm)

---

310. The only reliable method of ruling out pseudomyopia or accommodative spasm is with a cycloplegic drug, thus relaxing accommodation. If an emmetrope accommodates 2.00 D while viewing the 20 foot chart, what lens will be necessary to allow him to see the chart clearly while continuing to accommodate 2.00 D? (1) _____. To relax this accommodation (2) _____ may be necessary.

---

481. (1) divergent
(2) convergent

---

482. If, in retinoscopy, the lenses necessary to neutralize the reflex are $+1.00 - 2.00 \times 180$ and 66.66 cm is the working distance, the net retinoscopy will be _____.

653. (1) in (3) in

(2) diplopia (or (4) fusion (or single

double vision) vision

---

654. Any ametropia except latent hyperopia should be corrected when testing fusional reserves. When the divergence reserve at distance is tested accommodation should play no role, since any relaxation of accommodation will cause an increase in divergence fusional reserve. If accommodation played a role in divergence testing at distance, a patient's lenses did not have enough _____ power.

---

825. No

---

826. Despite the fact that patients who need a low reading add can accommodate sufficiently for clear intermediate vision, the absence of lines of demarcation on variable addition lenses offers some cosmetic advantages. Variable addition lenses are worn by early presbyopes primarily for _____ reasons.

---

997. 40

---

998. A 46-year-old lawyer needs a presbyopic correction of a $+1.25$ D add. The minimum add for the first bifocals is (1) _____ D, and the type bifocal recommended for this patient would be (2) _____ .

138. (1) +3.00

(2) 180

---

139. Transposition can be carried out as just described by diagram. The net result is

plano $- 3.00 \times 90 = -3.00 + 3.00 \times 180$.

The rules for changing from minus cylinder to plus cylinder expression are:

(1) Change the axis _____ degrees.
(2) Change the _____ of the cylinder.
(3) Algebraically _____ the old sphere and old cylinder to get the new sphere.

---

310. (1) -2.00 D

(2) a cycloplegic drug

---

311. The sudden appearance of myopia in a young adult is likely to be pseudomyopia or accommodative spasm. The onset of myopia at a yet older age usually heralds the developing cataract; as the nucleus of the lens becomes sclerosed the refractive power increases.

When a patient, age 60, notes he can now read without the aid of his glasses there is a strong possibility that the patient has _____ .

---

482. $-0.50 - 2.00 \times 180$

---

483. When you have noted the major axes with the handle of the retinoscope in the up position, neutralize one meridian, then the other. An easy method is to neutralize the meridian which is most minus (the one requiring the strongest plus lens) with a plus sphere. Then, keeping that lens in place neutralize the other principle meridian with a minus cylinder (axis parallel to the streak). Regardless of the working distance the power of the cylinder will be the same.

In the above method the meridian with the most minus power is neutralized with sphere and the other meridian with _____ cylinder.

654. plus (or convex)

---

655. As prism base in is increased, the eyes must diverge to maintain single vision. The amount of prism base in which just causes diplopia is a measure of the _____ fusional reserve.

---

826. cosmetic

---

827. For technical reasons, variable addition lenses are not useful for patients with large astigmatic errors and they also result in more aberrations than multi-focal lenses. Despite their theoretical advantages, therefore, they cannot be worn comfortably by all patients. A patient with 4.00 D of astigmatism needing a +1.25 D add for near (is/is not) a good candidate for variable addition spectacles.

---

998. (1) +1.25
(2) Executive (or other bifocal with a large segment)

---

999. If the 46-year-old male were a farmer instead of a lawyer, the bifocal type recommended would be (1) _____. The height of the bifocal should be (2) (higher/lower) in such an outdoor occupation.

139. (1) 90
   (2) sign
   (3) add

140. Write $+6.00 - 4.00 \times 80$ in plus cylinder form.

---

311. cataracts (and mild myopia)

312. The sudden development of myopia in a child will usually be true myopia; however, the danger is real that an increase in pressure (glaucoma) has caused the eye to elongate, thus producing the myopia.

The sudden development of myopia may herald conditions other than simple myopia, such as:

(1) _____ in children,
(2) _____ in young adults,
(3) _____ in adults.

---

483. minus

484. You found that (at a working distance of 66.66 cm) with the streak at 90 degrees a $+2.00$ D sphere neutralized the reflex; with the streak at 180 degrees (leaving a $+2.00$ D sphere in place) a -3.00 D cylinder neutralized the reflex.

The net retinoscopy is $+0.50 -$ _____ $\times 180$.

655. divergence

---

656. The amount of prism base in which just allows single vision to return after the break point has been determined indicates the recovery point. The closer the recovery point is to the break point the greater is the fusional reserve. Which patient has the greater fusional reserve?

Divergence fusional reserves
(Amplitudes of divergence)
Diplopia / Recovery

Patient A   16Δ B.I./12Δ B.I.
Patient B   16Δ B.I./ 4Δ B.I.

---

827. is not

---

828. Consider a 60-year-old emmetropic patient whose close work is generally at 33.33 cm. What add for near is necessary to have one-half of accommodation in reserve? (1) _____.
What add for intermediate distances is necessary? (2) _____.

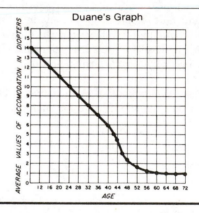

Duane's Graph

---

999. (1) any of the smaller bifocals such as Kryptok, Univis, or Full-Vu
    (2) lower

1000. The 46-year-old lawyer asks you if tints are advisable for his office wear. The eye rapidly adapts to small changes in brightness so a faint tint (would/would not) have any beneficial effect on an eye in the usual circumstances.

140. $+2.00 + 4.00 \times 170$

---

141. Neutralization of unknown lenses with trial lenses is tedious and inaccurate. An instrument which measures lenses by accurately noting the focal distance of lines is the Lensometer. The Lensometer measures spheres, cylinders, axes, and prisms. We suggest you find directions which accompany your Lensometer and, by experimentation with known lenses from your trial case, become competent in its use. Various automated lens measuring instruments are also available.

---

312. (1) glaucoma
(2) accommodative spasm (or pseudomyopia)
(3) cataracts

---

313. A transient myopia is frequently seen at the onset of diabetes mellitus and in diabetic acidosis. Anterior movement of the crystalline lens due to swelling of the ciliary body accounts for this. As the hyperglycemia is corrected the refractive error reverts to the original error. Many examiners prefer to wait two months after the patient's diabetes has been controlled before refracting the patient for permanent glasses.

If you checked a patient for glasses shortly after severe diabetes mellitus had been detected, too much (plus/minus) might be given the patient.

---

484. 3.00

---

485. You can use spheres to neutralize both axes. If in so doing you find that:

- with the streak at axis 45 degrees a -2.00 lens neutralizes the reflex,
- with the streak at axis 135 degrees, a $+5.00$ lens neutralizes the reflex,
- the gross retinoscopy is _____ $- 7.00$ $\times 45$.

(Remember that the streak parallels the axis of the cylinder.)

656. A

---

657. Base out prisms are used to measure convergence fusional reserve (or amplitude of convergence). Base out prism demands the eyes _____ to maintain single vision.

---

828. (1) +2.50 D (or +2.37 D)
  (2) +1.25 D (or +1.12 D)

---

829. If a patient has 1.00 D amplitude of accommodation, he will be able to work comfortably at distances between infinity and (1) _____
(leaving one-half of his accommodation in reserve). Through a +2.50 D add he will be able to work comfortably between 40 cm and (2) _____ .

An intermediate correction of +1.25 D add will enable him to work comfortably between 80 cm and (3) _____ (leaving one-half of his accommodation in reserve).

1000. would not

1001. The 46-year-old lawyer has heard of contact lenses. Would you recommend them instead of bifocals?

141. *(Advance to next frame.)*

---

142. A -5.00 D lens shows (1) _____
motion.

A $+1.00$ D lens shows (2) _____ motion and a (3) _____ lens shows no apparent motion.

---

313. minus $(-)$

---

314. The fovea of a myopic eye is situated slightly closer to the disc than the fovea of an emmetropic eye. Thus the visual axis projects slightly temporally from the center of the cornea. If this condition is marked, there is a small angle alpha and an apparent convergent squint may be noted. A myope may appear to have a mild convergent squint due to the relative location of the _____ .

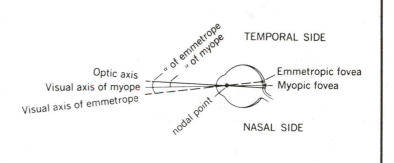

---

485. $+5.00$

---

486. You can use spheres to neutralize both axes. If in so doing you find that:

- with the streak at axis 90 degrees, a $+2.00$ lens neutralizes the reflex,
- with the streak at axis 180 degrees, a $+3.00$ lens neutralizes the reflex,
- the gross retinoscopy is $+3.00$ _____ $\times$ 90.

(Remember that the streak parallels the axis of the cylinder.)

657. converge

---

658. Convergence and accommodation are closely related. As the eyes accommodate they tend to converge. Esophoria is (greater/lesser) as accommodation is stimulated.

---

829. (1) 2 m
　　(2) 33.33 cm
　　(3) 57 cm

---

830. The height of a bifocal segment varies with the frame the patient selects. The optician will fit most bifocals so that the upper edge of the segment is 3 mm below the visual axis while the patient is fixating a distant object. An occasional patient will want only a small area superiorly for distance and the rest of the lens for near. For the average patient the upper edge of the bifocal segment should be (1) _____ below the (2) _____ .

1001. No (There are bifocal contact lenses, but these are not recommended for the usual case.)

1002. The 46-year-old lawyer plays tennis a great deal.

(1) Should a second pair of glasses for tennis be bifocals?
(2) If he desires a tinted glass for tennis should the tint be light or dark?
(3) Should the second pair be a safety glass?

142. (1) with
(2) against
(3) plano

143. Visual acuity is a measurement of the smallest retinal image the form of which can be recognized. Opacities in the eye and refractive errors may reduce acuity of an eye with an intact sensory system. A refractive error can be corrected by the appropriate combination of lenses. Opacities in an eye, however, cannot be corrected short of surgery and will cause a reduced _____ .

---

314. macula (or fovea or visual axis)

315. The choroid is frequently thinned around the myopic disc, allowing a white crescent of sclera to show through the retina. This crescent is called a myopic crescent. The photo shows such a crescent.

The photo is of a (1) _____ fundus with a (2) _____ disc.

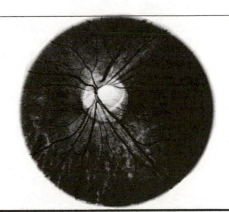

---

486. -1.00

487. You can use spheres to neutralize both axes. If in so doing you find that:

- with the streak at axis 45 degrees, a -1.00 lens neutralizes the reflex,
- with the streak at axis 135 degrees, a -3.00 lens neutralizes the reflex,
- the gross retinoscopy is $-1.00 - 2.00 \times$ _____ .

(Remember that the streak parallels the axis of the cylinder.)

658. greater

---

659. As prism base out is increased the eyes maintain single vision until the convergence reserve is exhausted. Accommodation is then utilized to elicit further convergence to maintain single vision. That convergence so elicited is called accommodative convergence (or accommodative fusional reserve). Base out prisms are increased until the 20/40 line blurs. This is the point at which the patient is beginning to accommodate and thus utilize _____ .

---

830. (1) 3 mm
   (2) visual axes (as the patient is fixating a distant object)

---

831. The strength of an unknown bifocal add can be measured by neutralization or with the lensometer. The _____ is the more exact of the two methods.

1002. (1) No
   (2) Dark
   (3) Yes

1003. A 16-year-old female complains of blurred vision. You find she needs − 1.75 D OD and − 2.25 D OS to give her 20/20 in each eye.

   A + 0.25 D over either eye blurs the 20/20 line. What is the prescription you would order?

143. visual acuity

---

144. The same sized object moved closer to the eye will cause a (1) _____ retinal image; the size of the object is, therefore, a poor way of measuring visual acuity unless the (2) _____ of the object from the eye is also stated.

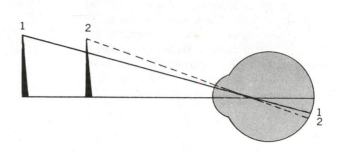

---

315. (1) myopic
(2) myopic crescent

---

316. Farsightedness or hypermetropia (synonymous with hyperopia) exists when parallel light rays entering the eye focus behind the eye. Just as the most frequent cause of myopia is axial, so it is that most hypermetropia is axial. Most hyperopic eyes are of _____ length than emmetropic eyes.

---

487. 135

---

488. You can use spheres to neutralize both axes. If in so doing you find that:

- with the streak at axis 45 degrees, a −0.50 lens neutralizes the reflex,
- with the streak at axis 135 degrees, a +2.50 lens neutralizes the reflex,
- the gross retinoscopy is _____.

(Remember that the streak parallels the axis of the cylinder.)

659. accommodative fusional reserve
(or accommodative convergence)

---

660. Base out prism is increased until the 20/40 line just starts to blur. The amount of this prism is recorded and measures the convergence (1) _____ at distance. Base out prism is increased until diplopia is reported. The amount of prism added from the point of blurring until diplopia is reported is a measure of the (2) _____.

---

831. lensometer

---

832. When using the lensometer the back vertex power is measured by having the convex side of the lens toward you. When the lens is reversed to bring the concave side toward you the _____ vertex power is measured.

1003. OD −1.75 D sphere
OS −2.25 D sphere

1004. The 16-year-old patient asks if her myopia of 1.75 D OD and 2.25 D OS (1) is hereditary and if so, (2) is it a dominant or recessive trait?

144. (1) larger
(2) distance

---

145. If the visual acuity is expressed in terms of the angle subtended by an object, then the distance the object is from the eye will be unimportant. The E's —E_1, E_2, and E_3—subtend _____ angles.

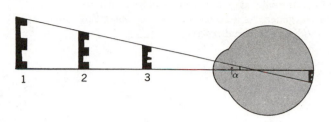

---

316. less (or shorter)

---

317. Total hypermetropia may be divided into latent and manifest. The manifest hyperopia may be further divided into absolute and facultative. The latent can only be measured with the use of a cycloplegic. To measure each of the above we first increase the power of the plus lenses until the best distance vision is attained; this final lens is a measure of the absolute hyperopia. Second, more plus is added until the next strongest lens decreases the vision. The difference between the first step and second step is a measure of (1) _____ hypermetropia. Third, a cycloplegic is given, and after a suitable period of time, more plus will be necessary to give the best vision; this additional plus measures the (2) _____ hypermetropia.

---

488. $+ 2.50 - 3.00 \times 45$
(or $-0.50 + 3.00 \times 135$)

---

489. You can use spheres to neutralize both axes. If in so doing you find that:

- with the streak at axis 45 degrees, a -2.00 lens neutralizes the reflex,
- with the streak at axis 135 degrees, a $+5.00$ lens neutralizes the reflex,
- the gross retinoscopy is _____.

(Remember that the streak parallels the axis of the cylinder.)

660. (1) fusional reserve (or amplitude)
     (2) accommodative fusion reserve
        (or accommodative convergence)

661. Accommodative fusional reserve is a measure of the accommodation which can be used to stimulate convergence. As accommodation decreases the accommodative fusional reserve _____.

832. front

833. If the distance portion of a bifocal is below 2.00 D simply measure the distance portion in the usual fashion with the lensometer (convex surface toward you), elevate the lens, and focus one set of lines through the center of the add. The difference in power between the reading of one set of lines focused through the distance and the same set of lines focused through the add is _____.

1004. (1) Yes
      (2) Dominant

1005. Just before the 16-year-old patient leaves your office you find that she was started on insulin one week ago. -1.75 D OD and -2.25 D OS gave her 20/20 in each eye. (1) What lens would you prescribe? (2) Why?

145. equal (or the same)

---

146. Visual acuity is usually measured as minimum separable acuity. Other visual acuity measurements include minimum visible and vernier acuity. The following test objects are for what visual acuity measurements?

(1)	(2)	(3)
.	‖	╷
With poorer vision no dot is seen.	With poorer vision one line is seen.	With poorer vision an unbroken line is seen.
(1)	(2)	(3)
_____ acuity	_____ acuity	_____ acuity

---

317. (1) facultative
(2) latent

---

318. As more plus is placed before a patient who continues to have no decrease in vision, we say "he accepts more plus." One method of getting a hyperope to accept more plus, thus measuring all of his facultative hypermetropia, is to first place such a great amount of plus lenses in place that the subject's vision is blurred to 20/400. This additional plus causes accommodation to relax. After a suitable time the plus is reduced 0.25 D at a time until the best vision is obtained. After the 20/100 line is reached each 0.25 D reduction will allow the subject to read about one line further down the vision chart. The purpose of blurring the hyperope with strong plus lenses is to _____.

---

489. $- 2.00 + 7.00 \times 135$
(or $+ 5.00 - 7.00 \times 45$)

---

490. If the gross retinoscopy is $+ 5.00 - 7.00 \times 45$ and the working distance is 66.66 cm, the net retinoscopy is _____.

661. decreases

662. The relation of accommodation to convergence in a given patient may be found by measuring the horizontal phorias before and after stimulating accommodation and noting the phoria change. This is done by having the patient read the 20/40 line wearing his distance correction, dissociating the eyes vertically with 6Δ base up, measuring the horizontal phoria, then placing a −1.00 D sphere OU over his correction and repeating the horizontal phoria measurement. The purpose of the minus 1.00 D sphere is _____.

---

833. the power of the add

834. The front vertex power is usually used to measure the add in fused bifocals when the distance correction is greater than 2.00 D. The front vertex power is slightly different from the back vertex power. The concave side (back of the lens) should be toward you when measuring the add of a

(1) _____ (2)_____.
    (type of bifocal)   (power of distance lens)

1005. (1) None
(2) Uncontrolled diabetes causes a change of the crystalline lens position. She may be an emmetrope when the diabetes is controlled.

1006. You know that the lens which gives 20/20 OD is a −1.75 D lens. (1) What retinoscopic reflex motion would you expect at 50 cm with no lenses before this eye? (2) What motion would you expect at 66.66 cm? (3) What lens would cause neutrality of the reflex at 50 cm?

146. (1) Minimum visible
(2) Minimum separable
(3) Vernier

147. The minimum separable acuity is thought to depend on stimulation of two cones which are separated by a nonstimulated cone. Since one cone in the macular region is 0.004 mm in diameter, as measured histologically, two images on the retina must be separated at least this amount to be seen as two. The above relationship has been confirmed experimentally and corresponds to an angle of approximately one minute. If two cones, separated by a cone, are stimulated, (1) _____ image(s) will be perceived and will be at least (2) _____ minute(s) apart.

318. relax accommodation
(to measure all of facultative hyperopia)

319. Placing enough plus lenses before an eye to reduce visual acuity is called "fogging."

When the subject is fogged you have created an artificial (myopia/emmetropia/hyperopia).

490. $+ 3.50 - 7.00 \times 45$
(or $- 3.50 + 7.00 \times 135$)

491. Remember that the streak parallels the axis of the cylinder. If you find that:

- with the streak at axis 5 degrees, a $+1.00$ lens neutralizes the reflex,
- with the streak axis at 95 degrees, a $+5.00$ lens neutralizes the reflex, and working distance $=$ 66.66   cm,
- net retinoscopy is _____.

662. stimulation of 1.00 D of accommodation (to see its effect on phoria)

663. A 2Δ exophoria at distance might be changed to 1Δ esophoria with a minus 1.00 D sphere OU. This would give an accommodative convergence/accommodation ratio (ACA ratio) of 3Δ/1.00. The ACA ratio of −1.00 D changing a phoria of 2Δ exophoria to 2Δ esophoria would be _____ .

834. (1) fused
    (2) greater than 2.00 D

835. If the distance portion of a fused bifocal is greater than 2.00 D, the power of the add is derived from the front vertex powers of the two parts of the lens. Measure the distance portion in the usual fashion with the lensometer with the convex side of the lens toward you. Reverse the lens and focus one set of lines through the distance; raise the lens and focus the same set of lines through the center of the segment. This difference is the (1) _____ and is measured with the (2) (concave/convex) side of the lens toward you.

1006. (1) With
    (2) Against
    (3) +0.25 D

1007. To test the distant horizontal phoria without stimulating accommodation, you would use the (1) _____ to dissociate, (2) _____ to quantitate the phoria, and (3) _____ as the fixation point.

147. (1) two

   (2) one

---

148. The Snellen acuity chart, used for testing minimum separable acuity, is based on letters which are formed by lines one minute in width and separated by one minute. Such letters can be constructed for any test distance. The width of the entire letter E is _____ at the designated test distance.

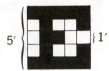

5′ ⎰⎱ ⎰ 1′

---

319. myopia

---

320. Hyperopia which cannot be compensated by the patient's accommodation is called absolute. If, upon placing plus lenses before an eye without cycloplegia, you find the patient reports better distance vision, he has measurable _____ hypermetropia. (Note that the term hyperopia can be used synonymously with hypermetropia.)

---

491. $+ 3.50 - 4.00 \times 5$

   $(- 0.50 + 4.00 \times 95)$

---

492. If you find that a $+2.00$ D sphere with a -2.00 D cylinder $\times 175$ degrees neutralizes all meridians at a working distance of 50 cm, the net retinoscopy is _____ .

663. $4\Delta/1.00$

664. ACA ratio is an abbreviation for _____ .

---

835. (1) power of the add
(2) concave

836.

PART XI

SPECTACLE ABERRATIONS

(Advance to next frame.)

1007. (1) Maddox rod
(2) prisms (revolving prisms)
(3) fixation light (at 20 feet)

1008. The Maddox rod should be placed (vertically/horizontally) to cause the patient to see a vertical line.

148. 5 minutes

---

149. The Snellen fraction is used to record visual acuity. A Snellen fraction of 20/40 means that at 20 feet a letter can be seen which is 5 minutes high and 5 minutes wide if measured at 40 feet. The numerator denotes the distance between patient and chart, and the denominator denotes the distance at which the width and height of the entire letter seen would subtend an angle of _____ .

---

320. absolute

---

321. An eye with its crystalline lens is called a phakic eye. If the crystalline lens of the eye is removed, as in a cataract operation, a severe form of hypermetropia is created. This is called aphakia.

Aphakia is corrected by strong _____ .

---

492. plano -2.00×175

---

493. If the pupil is widely dilated, you may note that the reflex in the periphery of the pupil will be opposite in motion to that in the central area of the pupil. This is caused by the difference in refractive power of the lens periphery. Only the central portion should be regarded in such an instance.

The _____ portion of the reflex is most significant.

664. accommodative convergence/accomodation ratio

665. If the ACA ratio is large, for example, 6Δ/1.00, you might expect excessive _____ at near.

---

836. (*Advance to next frame.*)

837. Knapp's rule states that when an axially ametropic eye (a long or short eye) is corrected by a lens placed at the anterior focal point of the eye, the magnification of the retinal image is equal to that of an emmetropic eye. Knapp's rule applies to axial astigmatism, but does it apply to the more common refractive astigmatism due to an aspheric cornea?

1008. horizontally

1009. An 8-year-old male is brought to you with the report that he failed the school vision test. You find:

$$\bigvee \begin{array}{ll} \text{OD } 20/70 & \text{P.H. } 20/30 \\ \text{OS } 20/80 & \text{P.H. } 20/30 - 3 \end{array}$$

The probable cause for his decreased vision is (a refractive error/a pathological condition).

149. 5 minutes

---

150. Snellen acuity is measured by noting how far down a patient can read on a Snellen chart placed at 20 feet. The right eye of the patient is occluded, and the patient reads E FP TOZ LPED PECFD ED. From Figure 1 in the Appendix note that the patient correctly read all of the 20/40 line and 2 of the 20/30 line. This is recorded as:

$$V_{OS} = 20/40 + 2$$

With the left eye occluded, he reads E FP TOZ LPED PECFD EDFCZP FE, which is recorded as:

$$V_{OD} = \underline{\hspace{2cm}}.$$

(See Fig. 1, p. 347.)

---

321. plus lenses

---

322. The eye has a total power of about +60.00 D, 40.00 D of which is due to the cornea and 20.00 D to the lens. Since we correct the aphakia with a spectacle lens much more anterior to the retina than the original crystalline lens, we can use a spectacle lens of longer focal length or a (stronger/weaker) lens than the original +20.00 D.

---

493. central

---

494. Occasionally glaring reflexes from the trial lenses plus artifacts from the eye will not allow you to see the reflex sufficiently clearly even if you retinoscope slightly off the visual axis. If this is the case, shorten the working distance. This will brighten the reflex and will only reduce accuracy slightly.

A shorter working distance _____ the reflex.

665. convergence (or esophoria)

---

666. If the ACA ratio is large, a large amplitude of convergence will be found due to the accommodation stimulating relatively large amounts of (1) _____ and thus maintaining (2) _____ against more base out prism.

---

837. No

---

838. The anterior focal point of the eye is about 15 mm anterior to the cornea. If a spherical correction is placed at this point before an axially ametropic eye, what will be the size of the retinal image compared to that in an emmetropic eye?

1009. a refractive error

1010. Retinoscopy of the 8-year-old without cycloplegia reveals a gross retinoscopy of:

OD + 3.00 − 2.00 × 180
OS + 3.50 − 2.00 × 180

The working distance was 66.66 cm. What is the net retinoscopy?

150. 20/30 + 2

151.

$$V \quad \begin{array}{l} OD = 20/30 \\ OS = 20/40 + 2 \end{array}$$

In this notation **V** means visual acuity, OD means oculus dexter or right eye, OS means oculus sinister or left eye. 20/40 + 2 means that the patient can read all of the 20/40 line and _____ letters on the next smaller line.

---

322. weaker (about 10.00 D)

---

323. If an intraocular plastic lens is placed in an eye, it is termed pseudophakic and is approximately emmetropic. An aphakic eye has (1) _____ lens, is (2) (myopic/hyperopic), and has (3) (normal/no) accommodation.

---

494. brightens

---

495. "Scissors motion" consists of two band reflexes which seem to cross as blades of scissors. This scissors motion will be occasionally noted, particularly if there has been corneal scarring. If noted, strive for neutrality in the center of the cornea. Even with this annoying reflex, the difference between with and against can usually be noted.

If aberrant reflexes are present, you will try to obtain neutrality over what area of the cornea (or pupil)?

666. (1) convergence
(2) fusion (or single vision)

---

667. Will the ACA ratio affect the divergence reserves at distance?

---

838. The same as (or equal to)

---

839. The rule which states that a lens placed at the anterior focal point of an eye which is axially ametropic produces no change in the size of the retinal image compared with an emmetropic eye is called _____ rule.

1010. OD + 1.50 − 2.00 × 180
OS + 2.00 − 2.00 × 180

1011. The net retinoscopy findings of a child who has never worn glasses are OD + 1.50 − 4.00 × 180 and OS + 2.00 − 4.00 × 180. These findings are confirmed by the cross cylinder test. The best vision attained with varying spheres is 20/30 OD and 20/30 − 1 OS.

(1) What is the probable cause of the decreased vision?
(2) Can the corrected vision be expected to improve?

151. 2

---

152. The object of visual acuity recordings is to document exactly how many letters the patient correctly identifies. If the patient misses one-half of a line of letters, either that line or the previous line can be recorded. As an example the decision to record $20/40 - 2$ or $20/50 + 3$ is usually made in favor of $20/40 - 2$ if there are five test letters in the $20/40$ line. Either notation is correct. With OS covered (wearing correction), the patient reads E FP TBE and with OD covered, he reads E FP TOZ LPED PBCBD. This is recorded as:

$$V_{*cc} \quad \begin{array}{l} OD = \underline{\hspace{2cm}} \\ OS = \underline{\hspace{2cm}} \end{array}$$

*with correction

(See Fig. 1.)

---

323. (1) no (no crystalline)
(2) hyperopic
(3) no

---

324. Most eyes are hyperopic by 2.50 to 3.00 D at birth. Well over 50 percent maintain hyperopia all their lives. Most adults will be (myopic/ hyperopic/emmetropic).

---

495. Center

---

496. With the retinoscope handle in the up position giving (1) _____ rays, against motion implies more (2) _____ is necessary and with motion implies more (3) _____ is necessary for neutrality.

667. No

---

668. The ACA ratio affects the divergence reserves at near, since accommodation can be relaxed permitting more base _____ prism to be overcome at near than at distance with fusion maintained.

---

839. Knapp's

---

840. The anterior focal point of the eye is about _____ mm in front of the cornea.

1011. (1) Astigmatism (previously uncorrected astigmatism, or refractive amblyopia) (2) Yes (with the constant use of the astigmatic correction)

1012. The refractive error of an 8-year-old patient is OD + 1.50 − 2.00 × 180 and OS + 2.00 − 2.00 × 180 as determined on the postcycloplegic refraction. What should be the final lens prescription? (Patient has no muscle imbalance.)

152. V $_{cc}$ OD 20/100 + 1
OS 20/40 − 2

153. The principle of a pinhole box camera is also used in measurement of visual acuity. The pinhole allows only the rays that are not refracted to enter the camera; thus no lenses are needed. We can eliminate most refractive errors of the eye with the same technique: have the patient read the Snellen chart through a pinhole. If poor vision is not improved with a pinhole, suspicion is aroused that the defective vision is not due to a _____.

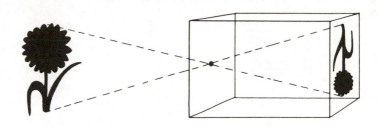

324. hyperopic

325. Low degrees of hyperopia are corrected by utilizing accommodation. Hyperopes, therefore, exert (1) (more/less) accommodation at distance and (2) (more/less) accommodation at near than emmetrope.

496. (1) divergent
(2) minus (or concave power)
(3) plus (or convex power)

497. A retinoscope with a line filament and line image capable of emitting either convergent or divergent rays is called a _____ retinoscope.

668. in

---

669. If a patient is orthophoric at distance and 18Δ esophoric at near, and has an ACA ratio of 6Δ/1.00, _____ lenses at near will decrease the accommodation required at near and decrease the esophoria at near.

---

840. 15

---

841. A spectacle lens worn 15 mm from the cornea is at the _____ focal point of the eye.

1012. OD + 1.50 − 2.00 × 180
OS + 2.00 − 2.00 × 180

1013. Federal law requires all glasses to be impact resistant. Plastic is ideal except for the cost and the easy manner in which the lenses become scratched. The more practical method of providing impact resistant glasses for children (except for high myopia) is by case-hardening glass. Case-hardening is a tempering process which hardens the lens surface.

   The most practical type of lenses for an 8-year-old is _____ and should be so indicated on the prescription.

153. refractive error

---

154. A patient who reads 20/40 s̄c (without correction and reads 20/20 P.H. (pinhole) probably has a _____ to explain the reduced visual acuity.

---

325. (1) more
    (2) more

---

326. Shortening of the eye may occur pathologically with tumors pressing on the back of the eye, tumors under the retina, swelling of the retina, detachment of the retina, and exudates under the retina. This would result in the development of

_____.
  (type of refractive error)

---

497. streak

498.

PART VII

SUBJECTIVE METHODS OF VERIFYING RETINOSCOPY

(Advance to next frame.)

669. plus

---

670. If the ACA ratio is $6\Delta/1.00$, then a $+1.50$ D add OU at near can be expected to change 12Δ esophoria at near to 3Δ E' (esophoria at near). For each 1 D of plus, 1 D of accommodation is relaxed and hence 6Δ of convergence is abolished. So for 1.50 D of plus, 9Δ convergence is abolished and the phoria changes from 12Δ E' to 3Δ E'.

If the ACA ratio is $4\Delta/1.00$, then a $+2.00$ D add OU at near can be expected to change an 18Δ esophoria at near to _____.

---

841. anterior

---

842. The refractive error of an aphakic eye (is/is not) mainly axial.

1013. case-hardened

1014. If you indicate on the prescription how well the patient can see with each eye, the optician can grossly verify the correctness of lenses with this information.

If a patient has the best correctable vision of 20/20 OD and 20/80 OS, it (is/is not) advisable to so note on the prescription to the optician.

154. refractive error

---

155. OD with glasses reads E FP TOZ LPED and with pinhole reads PECFD EDFCZP.

OS with glasses reads E FP TOZ and with pinhole reads LPED PECFD EDFCZP.

Vision is recorded as:

$$V_{cc} \quad \begin{array}{l} OD \text{\underline{\hspace{2cm}}} P.H. \text{\underline{\hspace{2cm}}} \\ OS \text{\underline{\hspace{2cm}}} P.H. \text{\underline{\hspace{2cm}}} \end{array}$$

(See Fig. 1.)

---

326. hyperopia

---

327. The chief complaint of a hyperope will depend principally upon the amount of hyperopia and accommodation present. (Special conditions such as strabismus will be considered later.) If absolute hyperopia is present, the patient's uncorrected near and distant vision will be (1) _____. By definition absolute hyperopia is the hyperopia which the eye's (2) _____ cannot compensate.

---

498. *(Advance to next frame.)*

---

499. An 18-year old patient (patient A) complains of poor distance vision and wears no glasses. On vision testing, the patient reads

OD—E, FP, TCZ; P.H.— E, FP, TOZ, LPED, PECFD, EDRCZF

OS—E, FF; P.H.— E, FP, TOZ, LPED, PEORD

(See Fig. 1.)

The visual acuity is OD (1) _____, P.H. (2) _____; OS (3) _____, P.H. (4) _____.

(Record the visual acuities on the data sheet for future reference. See Fig. 7, p. 353.)

670. 10Δ E' (esophoria at near)

---

671. Exophoria means the eyes turn (1) _____
when fusion is interrupted and is measured with
prism base (2) _____ .

---

842. is not

---

843. Magnification of a retinal image is positive if
the image size is increased and negative if it is
decreased in comparison to that in an emmetropic
eye. A minus lens which reduces retinal image size
compared to an emmetropic eye is producing
_____ magnification.

1014. is

1015. A 6-year-old male is brought to you with the
report that his eyes have turned in intermittently
for the past two years.
   What cycloplegic drug (1) _____
                              (drug and percentage)
should be used (2) _____ ?
                   (frequency and for how long)

155. V_{cc} OD 20/50 P.H. 20/30
OS 20/70 P.H. 20/30

156. OD without glasses reads E FP TOZ LPED PECFD EDFCZP and with pinhole shows no improvement.

OS without glasses reads E FP TOZ LPED PECFD EDFCZP and with pinhole shows no improvement.

This is recorded as _____. *(See Fig. 1.)*

---

327. (1) blurred
(2) accommodation

328. If the volume of near work increases, a patient previously comfortable may complain of eye strain. This is usually manifested by dull discomfort about the eyes, burning of eyes, tearing, and a mild headache occasionally accompanied by periodic failure of accommodation and consequent blurring of vision.

In many instances the patient will tolerate these symptoms. Frequently the discomfort demands help. In such instances the total hyperopia must be measured. This can only be determined with the use of a _____.

---

499. (1) 20/70 − 1   (2) 20/30 − 2
(3) 20/200 + 1   (4) 20/40 − 2
(or 20/100^{-1})

500. The P.D. of patient A measures approximately 62 mm. The patient's face is fairly symmetrical so the lens carrier before each eye is set at

_____.

671. (1) out

(2) in

---

672. Esophoria means the eyes turn (1) _____ when fusion is interrupted and is measured with prism base (2) _____ .

---

843. negative

---

844. Correction of ametropia due to refractive aberrations in the eye produces _____ of the retinal image compared to that in an emmetropic eye.

1115. (1) atropine ointment 0.5 percent   or   (1) 1 drop each of proparacaine, 2 percent

(2) 1 time a day for 3 days prior   cyclopentolate, and 1 percent tropicamide

to refraction   (2) 1 time 20 minutes prior to refraction

1016. Retinoscopy of the 6-year-old shows gross findings of OD + 7.00 − 1.00 × 180 and OS + 7.00 − 1.00 × 180 at working distance of 50 cm.

The net retinoscopy is (1) _____ . This is astigmatism (2) _____ the rule.

156. $\underset{sc}{V}$ OD 20/30 P.H. 20/30
_{sc} OS 20/30 P.H. 20/30

157. A patient with amblyopia ex anopsia (reduced vision from disuse) exhibits poor vision. The patient will usually be able to read several lines better if one letter at a time is presented. A patient with a constantly deviating left eye might read

OD: FP TOZ LPED PECFD EDFCZP FELOPZD DEFPOTEC and with OS: E FP TOZ. P.H. same. Using isolated letters the patient might read the next two lines LPED PECFD.

This would be recorded:

$\underset{sc}{V}$ OD _____

_{sc} OS _____ P.H. _____

Isolated

letter _____

(See Fig. 1.)

---

328. cycloplegic drug

329. A patient using more than one-half of his amplitude of accommodation for a visual task can be expected to have symptoms of eye strain. An uncorrected hyperope of 2.00 D will require a total of 5.00 D accommodation to see clearly at 33.33 cm. If he has an amplitude of accommodation of 7.50 D, you can allow him to use only 3.75 D (50% of 7.50 D). How much plus will you have to prescribe for his work at 33.33 cm to leave 50 percent of his accommodation in reserve, thus relieving his symptoms?

---

500. 31 mm

501. With the P.D. set, the trial frame is placed on the patient and adjusted for (1) _____, (2) _____, and (3) _____.

672. (1) in
  (2) out

673. Crossed diplopia (after dissociation) indicates a patient has _____.

---

844. magnification (negative or positive)

---

845. A correction placed 12 mm from an axially ametropic eye (will/will not) change the magnification of the retinal image.

1016. (1) OD + 5.00 − 1.00 × 180
      OS + 5.00 − 1.00 × 180
    (2) with

1017. During the first visit the patient's eyes deviated nasally approximately 30Δ when either eye was covered. Since he is a 5.00 D hyperope you would expect that correction of the hyperopia would (1) (increase/decrease) the intermittent nasal deviation of the eyes (esophoria-tropia), by (2) (increasing/decreasing) the accommodative demands at near and distance.

157. V_{sc} OD 20/20
OS 20/70 P.H. 20/70 Isolated letter 20/40

---

158. The ability of amblyopes to read isolated letters better than full lines is so characteristic that other conditions should be carefully looked for when an amblyope does not show this characteristic. The patient has a right exotropia and reads with OD cc E FP TOZ, pinhole, no improvement, and isolated letters TOZ LPED. The patient reads cc DEFPOTEC with OS.

The vision is recorded as: (1) _____ .

The patient shows improvement in vision OD with isolated letters. The diagnosis of (2) _____ is probably correct. *(See Fig. 1.)*

---

329. +1.25 D

---

330. Low hyperopia (below 6.00 D) is usually a dominant trait (as in low myopia). High degree of hyperopia, again as with myopia, is usually a recessive trait (100 percent of children will be affected if both parents have high hypermetropia).

Ho	*Hh*	*hh*	*ho*	*oo*
low	low	high	emmetrope	emmetrope
hyperope	hyperope	hyperope	(carrier)	(noncarrier)

If one parent is a high hyperope and the other parent an emmetrope (a noncarrier) then (none/50 percent/all) of their children would be expected to have high hyperopia.

---

501. (1) temple length
(2) pantoscopic tilt } in any order
(3) nose shape

---

502. When cycloplegia is not used with retinoscopy, the patient's accommodation must be relaxed. The relaxation may be accomplished with plus lenses over the fixating eye to fog the patient (with the use of any distant fixation object) or by utilizing a distant fixation light which does not stimulate accommodation. When neither plus lenses nor cycloplegia are used during retinoscopy, the patient is instructed to fixate on _____ .

673. exophoria

---

674. Uncrossed diplopia (after dissociation) indicates a patient has _____.

---

845. will

---

846. Minus lenses decrease and plus lenses increase the size of retinal images unless Knapp's rule is effective. In mixed astigmatism the magnification in the meridian with plus power is (1) (positive/negative) and in the meridian with minus power (2) (positive/negative).

1017. (1) decrease
　　　(2) decreasing

1018. Since the aim of a hyperopic correction, when the patient has an accommodative esophoria-tropia, is to relieve as much accommodation as possible, we correct (all/none) of the latent hyperopia.

158. (1) V OD 20/70 P.H. 20/70 Isolated letters 20/50
cc OS 20/20

(2) amblyopia ex anopsia

159. Attention to the pattern in which a patient reads a chart will frequently give a clue to an unsuspected diagnosis. If a patient has trouble with the first few letters of each line, but reads the remainder of each line correctly, left hemianopsia (blindness of the left visual field) should be suspected. The patient has difficulty locating the start of the next line each time. If the patient reads "E L, no FP, O, no TOZ, E, no P, no LPED" OD, and OS "EFP Z, no O, no TOZ, E, no P, no LPED, E, no PE CFD", then (1) _____ (2) _____

                 (side)   (type)

visual field defect should be suspected. *(See Fig. 1.)*

---

330. none

---

331. Hyperopic eyes frequently have an optic disc which appears to be slightly elevated as in papilledema, but there are no other signs of increased intracranial pressure, such as venous distention or hemorrhages.

   This is called pseudopapilledema of hyperopia.

   The photo shows such a disc. The photo is of a (1) _____ fundus with (2) _____ of the disc.

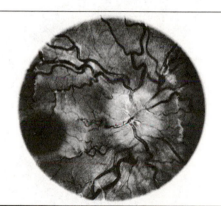

---

502. the distant fixation light

---

503. Retinoscopy should be done as nearly along the patient's visual axis as possible. When the patient is directed to fixate on a distant point, the retinoscope is held in the examiner's right hand and the examiner's right eye is used to retinoscope the patient's right eye. Under these circumstances the patient is maintaining fixation with his left eye. This procedure permits retinoscopy along the _____ of the patient's right eye.

674. esophoria

---

675. Near phorias are measured at 14 inches in the same manner as distance phorias. Dissociation of the eyes is necessary, followed by the use of prisms (preferably revolving) to align the images. Near phorias are measured at _____.

---

846. (1) positive
(2) negative

---

847. Axial changes are not responsible for all ametropia, astigmatism is never axial in healthy eyes, and most corrections are worn closer to the eyes than 15 mm. In most instances spectacles (do/do not) produce magnification of retinal image.

1018. all

1019. After the patient has worn the $+5.00 - 1.00 \times 180$ O U continuously for 6 weeks, we find that his eyes are straight, and the parent reports they are straight as long as he wears the glasses. The esophoria-tropia is _____ in origin.

159. (1) left
(2) hemianopsia

160. A right hemianopsia will usually cause the patient to have difficulty advancing to the next letter, and he will tend to repeat letters he has read.

A patient that reads OD cc "E FF P T – TO – TOZ LP LPED PE – PECF PECFD," OS cc "E FP T – T – TOZ LP – LPE LPED PE PEC PECFD" may have a _____. *(See Fig. 1.)*

331. (1) hyperopic
(2) pseudopapilledema

332. Many surfaces, such as those of doughnuts and tires, are not spherical but toric, thus having maximum and minimum radii of curvature. The inside of a teaspoon could be said to have a concave toric surface and the back of a teaspoon to have a convex toric surface. When such toric surfaces are involved in refracting surfaces, astigmatism is the result.

A lens with a spherical back surface and a toric front will produce _____.

503. visual axis

504. When a patient is directed to fixate on a distant object for retinoscopy, the patient's left eye is retinoscoped by the examiner's (1) _____ eye while the examiner holds the retinoscope in his (2) _____ hand.

675. 14 inches (33.33 cm)

---

676. If a fixation light is used as the target for phoria measurements at near, what method is best to disrupt fusion and dissociate the eyes?

---

847. do

---

848. Unequal refractive state in the two eyes is known as anisometropia. In anisometropia the magnification of retinal images will be _____ in the two eyes unless Knapp's rule is effective in each eye.

1019. accommodative

1020. Eight weeks after removing cataracts from a 65-year-old male the eyes are white and quiet. The net retinoscopy is:

OD + 12.00 − 1.00 × 90
OS + 11.50 − 1.00 × 90

The retinoscopy is correct. What is the final prescription for distance?

160. right hemianopsia

---

161. Numbers can be drawn similar to Snellen letters—the width of each line is 1 minute and the separation of the lines is 1 minute. Snellen numbers are quite helpful in patients who do not read English well. With OD cc the patient reads 85 293 8754 63952 428356 3746285 7264793; with OS cc he reads 85 239 8754 68662. P.H. 63952 428356 3746285 7264793 3876387. This would be recorded as:

$$V_{cc} \quad \begin{matrix} OD \underline{\hspace{2cm}} \\ OS \underline{\hspace{2cm}} \end{matrix}$$
(number chart)

(See Fig. 2, p. 348.)

---

332. astigmatism (or a cylindrical lens)

---

333. Just as different radii of curvature on a refracting surface produce an astigmatic error in any optical system, so will different radii on the surface of the cornea produce the condition called astigmatism.

If the radii of the cornea are converted to diopters and we find the 90 degree meridian to measure 44.00 D and the 180 degree meridian 40.00 D, this eye may have an (1) _____ error of (2) _____ D.

---

504. (1) left
    (2) left

---

505. To obtain a true axis of astigmatism of any eye, either using retinoscopy or subjective tests, the patient's head must be kept erect. A tilt of the patient's head to the left will result in a clockwise rotation of the axis of astigmatism from the observer's point of view. This rotation can be corrected by _____ the patient's head.

676. Maddox rod

---

677. What is the best means of dissociation if you wish to have accommodation stimulated and controlled by means of a reduced Snellen chart while testing the horizontal near phoria?

---

848. unequal (or different)

---

849. A patient needing a $+2.00$ D correction OD and -2.00 D correction OS is said to have _____ in describing his unequal refractive state.

1020. OD $+ 12.00 - 1.00 \times 90$
OS $+ 11.50 - 1.00 \times 90$

1021. The trial frame with the correction of:

OD $+ 12.00 - 1.00 \times 90$
OS $+ 12.00 - 1.00 \times 90$

is 15 mm from the eye, but the patient's glasses fit 10 mm from his eye. What is the final lens (sphere and cylinder) required OU (to nearest 1/8 D)? (Each meridian must be calculated separately.)

161. OD 20/20

OS 20/70 + 2 P.H. 20/20 + 3

---

162. When neither numbers nor letters can be read, as in the case of preschool children and illiterates, the tumbling E Chart can be used. The patient is asked to indicate the direction of the E with his hand. A parent can teach this "E game" to the child before the office visit. The child responds:

OD$_{sc}$ ◄ ↑ ◄ ➤ ◢◣   continuing on down

OS$_{sc}$ ◄ ↑ ◄ ➤ ◢ ◣   the chart

P.H. ◄ ↑ ◄ ➤ ┃ ➤ ➤ ◢◣

P.H. ◄ ↑ ◄ ➤ ┃ ➤ ➤ ◢◣

Note that the child gets all of the 20/70 line correct except for one E with the left eye. With pinhole he misses only one letter of the 20/30 line with each eye. This would be recorded as:

$$V_{sc} \quad \begin{array}{l} OD = \underline{\hspace{2cm}} \\ OS = \underline{\hspace{2cm}} \end{array} \quad \textit{(See Fig. 3, p. 349.)}$$

Es

---

333. (1) astigmatic

(2) 4.00

---

334. Any toric surface has maximum and minimum radii of curvature—usually 90 degrees apart. As a result, we can consider any toric surface to have a spherical component with a cylindrical component added. A cornea with a power of 42.00 D at 180 degrees and 43.00 D at 90 degrees could be considered as having a spherical component of (1) _____ D and (2) _____ D cylinder.

---

505. straightening

---

506. Gross retinoscopy of patient A at a working distance of .66 m results in the following findings:

OD + 0.50 − 1.00 × 30

OS + 0.50 − 1.50 × 180

The net, or corrected, retinoscopy OD is (1) _____ and OS (2) _____ (use minus cylinders). Record these findings on the data sheet. *(See Fig. 7.)*

677. Vertical prism (about 6Δ)

---

678. Since accommodation stimulates convergence, an uncorrected hyperope would be expected to show (1) _____, and plus lenses would
(what phoria)
be expected to (2) (reduce/increase) that phoria.

---

849. anisometropia

---

850. A difference in image size or shape between the two eyes is known as aniseikonia. A small physiological aniseikonia is a helpful clue to stereopsis and results from the lateral separation of the eyes. One stereopsis clue is based on physiologic _____ .

1021. $+12.75 - 1.12 \times 90$

1022. You determine that an aphakic patient's usual working distance is 14 inches. The necessary bifocal add is _____ D.

162. OD 20/70 P.H. 20/30 − 1
OS 20/70 − 1 P.H. 20/30 − 1

---

163. Landolt rings are similar to the tumbling E's since the patient simply has to indicate where the 1 minute break is in the Landolt ring. The patient indicates the direction of the ring opening with his hand as follows:

Note that the patient gets the 20/100 rings correct and one ring on the 20/70 line correct. With pinhole, all but one ring on the 20/50 line is correct. *(See Fig. 4, p. 350.)*

ODcc ◖ ◢ ◣ ◢ ◣ ◢   P.H. ◗ ◢ ◣ ◣ ◢ ◖◗ ◖◗ ◣ ◢
OS—No light perception.

Recorded as: $\mathbf{V}$ $\dfrac{\text{ODcc}\rule{4cm}{0.4pt}}{\text{OS}\quad \text{No L.P.}}$

---

334. (1) 43.00   (1) 42.00
(2) −1.00   (2) +1.00

---

335. If the powers of two meridians are different, their focal distances will differ. Consider an eye: (Remember a cylinder produces a focal line parallel to its axis.)

The vertical axis (90 degrees from the meridian) has a focus (1) (in front of/behind) the retina; the horizontal axis has a focus (2) (in front of/behind) the retina and this eye is called an

(3) _____ eye.

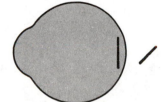

---

506. (1) −1.00 − 1.00 × 30
(2) −1.00 − 1.50 × 180

---

507. On the basis of retinoscopy the posterior focal line of the uncorrected conoid of Sturm within each eye of patient A is located _____ to the retina. *(Refer to data sheet; see Fig. 7.)*

678. (1) esophoria
(2) reduce

679. An uncorrected myope would be expected to show (1) _____ at near, since less accommo-
(phoria)
dation is used. The correct minus lenses would tend to (2) (increase/decrease) that phoria.

850. aniseikonia

851. A difference between the eyes in image size or shape is called _____.

1022. +3.00

1023. A patient who has had a cataract removed from one eye cannot tolerate the aniseikonia caused by a lens correcting the aphakia unless the correcting lens is a contact lens. As a result, the elderly patient is given no spectacle correction for his unilateral aphakic eye until the vision in his better eye fails. The elderly unilaterally aphakic patient has 20/30 vision in his phakic eye. Should an aphakic spectacle lens be given?

163. 20/100 + 1 P.H. 20/50 − 1
Landolt Rings

164. Children above three years can usually be taught the "E game." Have a parent cut out an E and practice with the child. A small box with E's of various sizes can also be used for teaching and testing. If a patient reads the 200 foot Snellen E at 8 feet his vision is 8/200. A patient could just make out the 100 foot Snellen E when you held it at 12 feet. This is expressed as: (OS was covered.)

OD = _____E Block

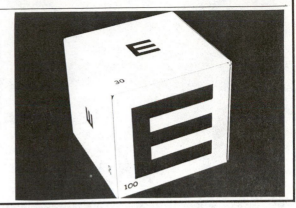

335. (1) in front of
(2) behind
(3) astigmatic

336. Astigmatism may be defined as that refractive state of an eye in which entering parallel rays of light fail to come to a point focus. If one of the meridians in astigmatism focuses on the retina, the condition is termed simple astigmatism. The site at which the other meridian focuses determines the condition to be either simple myopic astigmatism or simple hyperopic astigmatism. (A) is termed _____; (B) is termed _____.

507. anterior

508. On the basis of retinoscopy, patient A has the type of refractive error called _____ astigmatism in each eye. *(Refer to data sheet; see Fig. 7.)*

679. (1) exophoria
(2) decrease

680.

PART IX

PRESCRIPTION OF GLASSES

(*Advance to next frame.*)

---

851. aniseikonia

---

852. Aniseikonia may be optical or anatomical in nature. If optical, it may be inherent, depending on the difference between the dioptric systems of the eyes. It may also be acquired, if optical, resulting from the correcting lenses worn. Anisometropia can be expected to produce acquired _____ aniseikonia.

1023. No

1024. A refraction as part of a complete eye examination usually follows a set sequence. After the salient features of the history are reviewed, the visual acuity is measured. _____ visual acuity is then measured to ascertain that any reduced acuity is not due to disease.

165.

PART II

ACCOMMODATION

(Advance to next frame.)

---

336. (A) simple hyperopic astigmatism
(B) simple myopic astigmatism

---

337. If parallel rays enter an astigmatic eye and both foci lie behind the retina the condition is called compound hyperopic astigmatism. If both foci are in front the condition is called _____ .

---

508. compound myopic

---

509. In order to produce a visual acuity of about 20/40 with the posterior focal line of the conoid of Sturm still anterior to the retina, the circle of least confusion in compound myopic astigmatism may need to be moved nearer the retina. This is accomplished by placing before such an eye a sphere of _____ sign.

680. (*Advance to next frame.*)

---

681. An 18-year-old patient should have about (1) _____ D accommodative amplitude with a resultant near point of accommodation of about (2) _____.

Duane's Graph

---

852. optical

---

853. A small number of patients have aniseikonia on an anatomical basis, probably due to a difference between the eyes in the density of retinal receptors. A patient with no refractive error who has aniseikonia is said to have _____ aniseikonia.

1024. Pinhole

1025. After pinhole vision has been determined retinoscopy is done. The retinoscopy findings are then subjectively verified when possible. Subjective verification of astigmatic errors can be done with either (1) _____ or (2) _____.

165. (*Advance to next frame.*)

---

166. By action of the ciliary muscles, the human lens can become more spherical. This change in shape of the lens results in increased (plus/minus) refractive power.

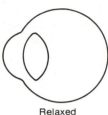 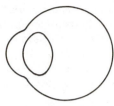

Relaxed   Accommodated

---

337. compound myopic astigmatism

---

338. Occasionally one focus will be in front, the other behind the retina. This is called mixed astigmatism. The diagrammed condition illustrates (1) _____ astigmatism. This refractive state could be corrected with a (2a) _____ sphere and a (2b) _____ cylinder, or a (3a) _____ sphere and a (3b) _____ cylinder.

 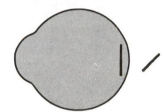

---

509. minus

---

510. An hyerope is considered overcorrected when he has too much plus. A myope is considered overcorrected when he has too much minus. An undercorrected myope has too _____ minus.

681. (1) 11.50

(2) 8.7 cm(± 1 cm)

---

682. As part of a refraction, the near point of accommodation is measured binocularly with the balanced distance correction in the trial frame. In this way the presence of presbyopia or accommodative spasm can be determined if a cycloplegic has not been used.

The presence of accommodative spasm or presbyopia can be detected by measuring the _____ .

---

853. anatomical

---

854. Aniseikonia may be symmetrical or asymmetrical. Symmetrical aniseikonia results in different sized retinal images. Asymmetrical aniseikonia results in different shaped retinal images. A difference in size of retinal images is present in _____ aniseikonia.

1025. (1) cross cylinders ⎫ either

(2) dials ⎭ order

1026. If accommodation must be minimized during refraction, the appropriate _____ drug is prescribed.

166. plus

---

167. The increase in plus power created by increased sphericity of the lens due to action of the ciliary muscles is termed accommodation. If accommodation is relaxed, plus power of the eye is (increased/decreased).

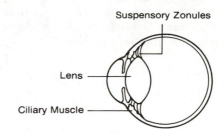

---

338. (1) mixed
(2a) plus (or convex) (2b) minus (or concave) } either
(3a) minus (3b) plus } order

---

339. If all the focusing lines, rather than only the two principal meridians, are considered, we would have two conical paths of light meeting at a circle in the center termed the circle of least confusion. At plane C the image of the point object will be the _____.

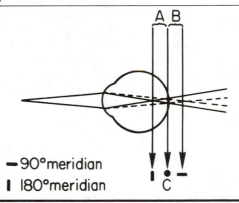

—90°meridian
I 180°meridian

---

510. little

---

511. A myopic patient is said to be fogged for the purpose of using astigmatic dials when the myopia is (undercorrected/overcorrected).

682. near point of accommodation

---

683. An 18-year-old patient requires minus lenses for clear distant vision. If, while wearing these minus lenses (without cycloplegia), his near point of accommodation is only 25 cm then _____ should be suspected.

---

854. symmetrical

---

855. Asymmetrical aniseikonia can only be anatomical or optically inherent. The images of optically acquired aniseikonia are different in size but the same in shape, hence optically acquired aniseikonia is termed _____.

1026. cycloplegic

1027. After the distance correction has been determined, the amplitude of accommodation is determined. Comfort doing near work requires that about _____ of accommodation be in reserve.

167. decreased

---

168. The amount of accommodation a human eye can exert is termed the amplitude of accommodation and is measured in diopters. An eye which can accommodate a total of 10.00 D has 10.00 D _____ of accommodation.

---

339. circle of least confusion

---

340. If the astigmatic error is small, then the circle of least confusion will be used by the patient as one desired "point" to focus on the retina. The circle of least confusion may be moved forward in the eye by the eye's own (1) _____, or by placing (2) _____ in front of the eye.

---

511. undercorrected

---

512. Astigmatic dials which have lines every 30 degrees are known as clock dials, and those having lines closer than every 30 degrees are known as fan type dials. An astigmatic dial with a line every 10 degrees is known as a _____ type dial.

683. accommodative spasm

---

684. Indications for cycloplegic refraction include accommodative spasm, youth, symptoms of hyperopia in the presence of insignificant manifest hyperopia on noncycloplegic refraction, strabismus, and difficulty in patient-physician communication. An 18-year-old patient suspected of accommodative spasm should have a _____ refraction.

---

855. symmetrical

---

856. Symmetrical aniseikonia may be overall or meridional. Overall symmetrical aniseikonia is caused by spherical differences in refraction. Anisometropia in one meridian as a result of unilateral high astigmatism can be expected to produce _____ symmetrical aniseikonia.

1027. 50 percent

1028. When the near and distance corrections have been tentatively made, the phorias are measured at (1) _____ and (2) _____ through these corrections.

168. amplitude

169. The closest distance to the eye at which an object remains clearly in focus is termed the near point of accommodation (NPA) and is the reciprocal of the amplitude of accommodation, expressed in meters. An eye with 10.00 D amplitude of accommodation has a near point of accommodation of $\dfrac{1}{\text{NPA}}$ = 10 D, NPA = 0.1 m or 10 cm.

If the patient's amplitude of accommodation is 5.00 D his near point of accommodation is _____ .

340. (1) accommodation
(2) plus lenses

341. The astigmatic eye depicted gives a line image at plane (1) _____ and plane (2) _____ .

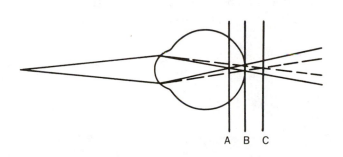

A B C

512. fan

513. If astigmatic dials are used, retinoscopy indicates the spherical lens which should be adequate for fogging, thus keeping the entire conoid of Sturm anterior to the retina. OD of patient A according to retinoscopy (would/would not) be fogged satisfactorily with a minus (−) 2.00 D sphere. *(Refer to data sheet; see Fig. 7.)*

684. cycloplegic

---

685. The younger the patient, the more the latent hyperopia, and the more effective the cycloplegic drug used must be. In children up to age 10 the classical cycloplegic drug of choice is _____ .

---

856. meridional

---

857. Spherical anisometropia can be expected to result in _____ symmetrical aniseikonia.

1028. (1) near ⎫ either
　　　　(2) distance ⎭ order

1029. The final prescription is based on the history, optical measurements, and the phoria measurements. If, after consideration of all the factors, a decision must be made to give a small correction versus no correction, usually give (the small/no) correction.

169. 20 cm (or 0.2 m)

170. The amplitude of accommodation is independent of the refractive error of the eye. It cannot be measured, however, unless the refractive error is corrected. For practical purposes, it is assumed that the emmetropic eye does not accommodate when viewing objects 20 feet (6 m) or more away. Before measuring the amplitude of accommodation the refractive error, if any, at _____ feet must be corrected.

341. A ⎱ either
 C ⎰ order

342. The conoid resulting from the different dioptric values of the principal meridians is called the conoid of Sturm. The images at the ends of the conoid of Sturm are (1) _____ and at the center a (2) _____ .

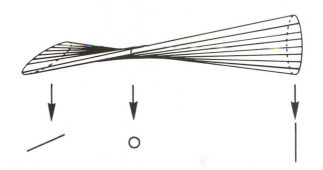

513. would not

514. The Lancaster-Regan astigmatic dial No. 1 has a spoke at every 10 degrees. Other types of dials have spokes every 15 or 30 degrees. If a patient sees several lines on any of these dials equally black and clear, the axis of the correcting minus cylinder is perpendicular to the middle line of this group. On the Lancaster-Regan dial No. 1 a patient reports the lines at 20, 30, and 40 degrees to be equally blacker and clearer than the others. The axis of the correcting minus cylinder is _____ degrees.

685. atropine

---

686. Systemic toxic effects may occur with the use of any cycloplegic. They include dry mouth, flushing, temperature elevation and temporary disorientation. Parents of children being given cycloplegics should be cautioned about the possible appearance of signs of _____.

---

857. overall

---

858. The instrument known as an eikonometer detects and measures aniseikonia. By means of polarization a different aspect of a target is presented to each eye, and the disparity in images is reported. The instrument used to measure aniseikonia is called an _____.

1029. no

1030. You are now a refractionist.

170. 20

---

171. To measure the amplitude of accommodation, the lens correcting the refractive error at 20 feet (distance correction) is placed before the eye. Print or test pattern is slowly brought closer to the eye, and the point at which the onset of blurring occurs is noted. The reciprocal of the distance (in meters) between the near point of accommodation and the eye is the amplitude of accommodation expressed as diopters. An emmetropic eye with a near point of accommodation of 12.5 cm (0.125 m) has an amplitude of accommodation of _____.

---

342. (1) lines
    (2) circle

---

343. The diagram demonstrates the conoid of (1) _____ with the circle of (2) _____ in the center.

---

514. 120

---

515. A −0.75 D sphere is placed in the back cell of the trial frame before the right eye of patient A, with an occluder in the frame before the left eye. The patient's visual acuity OD is now 20/40 − 1. The posterior focal line of the conoid of Sturm remains _____ to the retina according to the retinoscopy. *(See Fig. 7. Record −0.75 sphere on Figure 7 as fogging lens.)*

686. systemic toxicity

---

687. Patients over age 10 will generally have adequate cycloplegia following 1 percent cyclopentolate or 1 percent tropicamide. The duration of cycloplegia following either of these drugs is _____ compared to atropine, scopolamine, and homatropine.

---

858. eikonometer

---

859. Differences in image size over 5 percent are thought to be significant and produce symptoms indistinguishable from asthenopia of the usual origins. The image size difference in spectacle corrected monocular aphakia is about 33 percent. This (is/is not) sufficient to produce symptoms.

1030. *(Advance to go.)*

---

171. 8.00 D

---

172. It is possible to measure the amplitude of accommodation by determining the greatest minus lens which the eye (corrected for any error of refraction) can neutralize at 20 feet by accommodation. If vision at 20 feet begins to blur with a −4.00 D lens, the amplitude of accommodation is _____ .

---

343. (1) Sturm
(2) least confusion

---

344. If an astigmatic error is large, the patient may attempt to see using one of the linear foci, depending on the object under study. The patient may attempt to rid himself of all but one of the planes of light by squeezing his lids into a slit so only a horizontal plane of light enters the eye. If a patient looks through a fine slit he will eliminate his astigmatism and any remaining refractive error can be corrected by _____ lenses.

---

515. anterior

---

516. Degrees on the dials are marked to coincide with the degrees on the trial frame if the charts were superimposed on the patient's frame. In other words, a dial is a mirror image of the patient's frame. The degrees on the trial frame increase in a (1) (clockwise/counterclockwise) direction while the degrees in a dial increase in a (2) (clockwise/counterclockwise) direction.

687. short (brief)

---

688. Homatropine, which is used in concentrations of 2 percent and 5 percent, is the _____ effective of cycloplegic drugs.

---

859. is

---

860. Lenses which correct aniseikonia are called iseikonic lenses (or size lenses) and produce magnification either overall or meridionally without introducing refractive power. Aniseikonia is corrected by _____ lenses.

172. 4.00 D

(Return to Page 1, Frame 173.)

---

344. spherical

(Return to Page 1, Frame 345.)

---

516. (1) counterclockwise
(2) clockwise

(Turn to Page 2, Frame 517.)

688. least

(Return to Page 2, Frame 689.)

860. iseikonic (or size)

(Return to Page 2, Frame 861.)

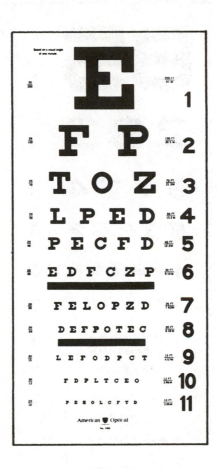

Figure 1
Snellen Letter Chart

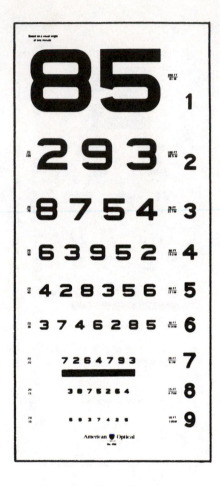

Figure 2
Snellen Number Chart

348

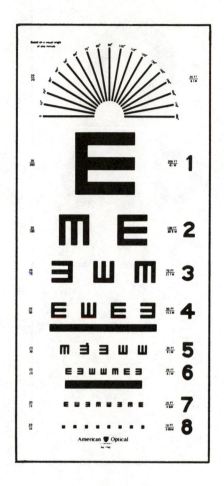

Figure 3
Snellen Illiterate E Chart

349

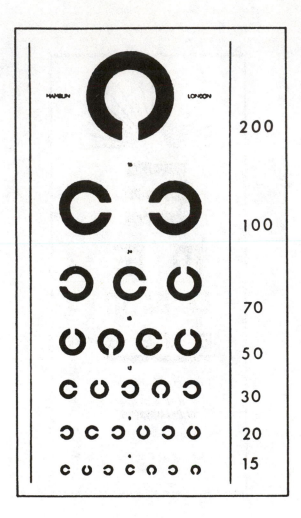

Figure 4
Landolt Ring Chart

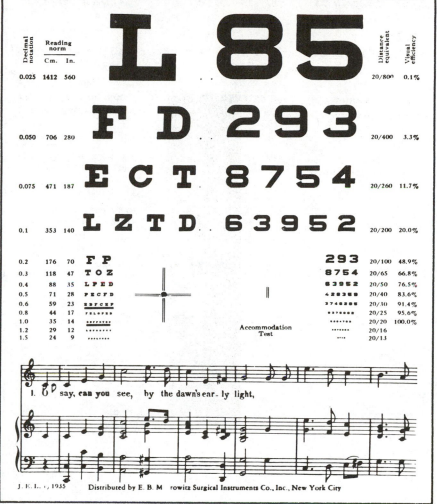

Figure 5
Lebensohn's Chart, Side 1

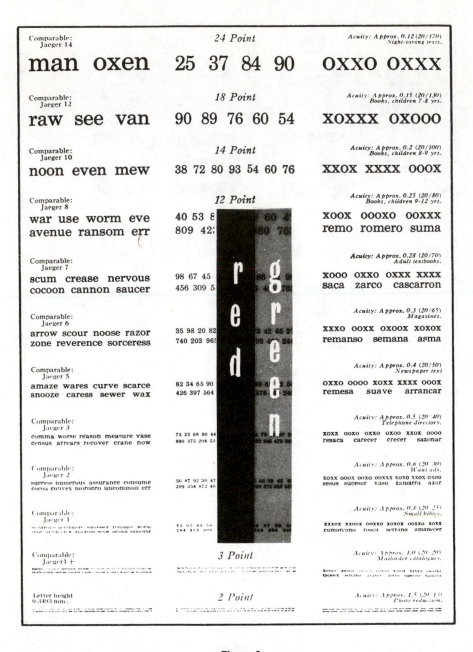

Figure 6
Lebensohn's Chart, Side 2

	OD	OS
Visual acuity	_____	_____
Pinhole vision	_____	_____
Net retinoscopy	_____	_____
Fogging lens	_____	_____
Working lens	_____	_____
Visual acuity with working lens in trial frames	_____	_____
Axis of astigmatism	_____	_____
Power of lenses with astigmatism only neutralized	_____	_____
Final correction	_____	_____

- -

	OD	OS
Visual acuity	_____	_____
Pinhole vision	_____	_____
Net retinoscopy	_____	_____
Fogging lens	_____	_____
Working lens	_____	_____
Visual acuity with working lens in trial frames	_____	_____
Axis of astigmatism	_____	_____
Power of lenses with astigmatism only neutralized	_____	_____
Final correction	_____	_____

- -

	OD	OS
Visual acuity	_____	_____
Pinhole vision	_____	_____
Net retinoscopy	_____	_____
Fogging lens	_____	_____
Working lens	_____	_____
Visual acuity with working lens in trial frames	_____	_____
Axis of astigmatism	_____	_____
Power of lenses with astigmatism only neutralized	_____	_____
Final correction	_____	_____

- -

	_____	_____

Figure 7

TABLE 1. CYCLOPLEGICS

	Procedure of Instillation	Time of Maximum Effect	Duration of Maximum Effect	Patient Able to Read	Accommodation Normal
Scopolamine HBr	2 drops 30 min apart	40 min after second drop	90 min	3 days	8 days
Cyclopentolate HCl (Cyclogyl)	2 drops 5 min apart	25 min after second drop	50 min	3 hr	18 hr
Atropine Sulfate Ointment	1 time daily for 3 days	18 hr after last instillation	8 – 24 hr	3 – 4 days	10 – 14 days
Tropicamide (Mydriacyl)	2 drops 5 min apart	20 min after second drop	15 min	45 min	4 hr
Homatropine HBr	6 – 8 drops 10 – 15 min apart	40 min after second drop	50 min	6 hr	36 hr
Combination: Proparacaine Tropicamide Cyclopentolate	1 drop each 30 sec apart	20 min after last drop	40 min	4 hr	24 – 48 hr

Index

Note: References in this index are to frame number, not to page number.